A Patient's Guide to Coronary Bypass Surgery and Its Aftermath

A Patient's Guide to Coronary Bypass Surgery and Its Aftermath

ADVICE FROM A SURVIVOR

Douglas C. Ewing

With an Introduction by Sir John Vane, FRS

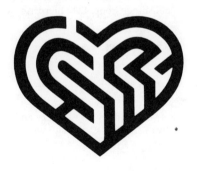

A BIRCH LANE PRESS BOOK
Published by Carol Publishing Group

To my son,

Douglas R. Ewing,

who casts his line straight and far and on his own mark

A Birch Lane Press Book
Published by Carol Publishing Group
Birch Lane Press is a registered trademark of Carol Communications, Inc.
Editorial Offices: 600 Madison Avenue, New York, N.Y. 10022
Sales and Distribution Offices: 120 Enterprise Avenue, Secaucus, N.J. 07094
In Canada: Canadian Manda Group, One Atlantic Avenue, Suite 105, Toronto, Ontario M6K 3E7
Queries regarding rights and permissions should be addressed to Carol Publishing Group, 600 Madison Avenue, New York, N.Y. 10022

Carol Publishing Group books are available at special discounts for bulk purchases, sales promotion, fund-raising, or educational purposes. Special editions can be created to specifications. For details, contact: Special Sales Department, Carol Publishing Group, 120 Enterprise Avenue, Secaucus, N.J. 07094

Manufactured in the United States of America
10 9 8 7 6 5 4 3 2 1

Library of Congress Cataloging-in-Publication Data

Ewing, Douglas C.
    A patient's guide to coronary bypass surgery and its aftermath : advice from a survivor / Douglas C. Ewing : with an introduction by Sir John Vane.
        p. cm.
    "A Birch Lane Press book."
    ISBN 1-55972-351-3 (hardcover)
    1. Coronary artery bypass—Popular works.   I. Vane, John R.   II. Title.
RD598.35.C37E94   1996
617.4'12—dc20   95-49372
                                                                 CIP

Contents

Foreword

When I met Douglas Ewing on the beautiful Caribbean island of Virgin Gorda at a cocktail party in 1993, his manuscript for this book was already largely completed. We had a lot to talk about, for we had both had bypass surgery, mine only a few months beforehand.

For most of my scientific life, I have been involved in research on the heart and blood vessels. As a pharmacologist, I have been fortunate to discover new concepts, new principles, and new drugs relating to arterial disease. Much of this work has been centered on the monolayer of cells that line all blood vessels, called the endothelial cells. These cells make all sorts of substances that help to keep the blood fluid. We discovered an important one of them in 1976 and called it prostacyclin. It prevents platelets from clumping together and also helps to keep the blood vessels open. Under a different name, prostacyclin was developed to the market as a treatment for peripheral vascular disease.

When I returned to academia in 1986, I started a research institute and named it after William Harvey, famed for his discovery of the circulation of blood, which was published in 1628 under the title "Exercitatio Anatomica de motu cordis et sanguinis in animalibus." The William Harvey Research Institute is a private foundation and now has over a hundred people working largely on the dysfunction of endothelial cells, which leads to arterial disease.

When I had bypass surgery in March 1992, unbeknownst to me (it would be, wouldn't it!) my surgeon took some pictures of my heart. Now when I lecture on the work we are doing, I show one of the pictures (a very gory one!) on the grounds that not many people can give a lecture on the cardiovascular system and illustrate it with a picture of their own heart.

I found Douglas Ewing's book very readable and informative, without being too scientific. It should be compulsory reading for those who have been told or know that they have increased risk factors for heart attacks; and many who have had coronary artery bypass graft (CABG) surgery (pronounced "cabbage"), will also find it fascinating, useful, and compelling. Families and friends of "cabbage" patients will also acquire a better understanding of the whole process, both before and after surgery, by dipping into this book.

JOHN VANE, FRS

Preface

I am not a doctor, nor indeed a scientist of any kind, and this is not a treatise on the technique or history of heart surgery. I had quadruple bypass surgery—known, if you haven't learned it yet, as "cabbage × 4"—the day before Thanksgiving 1986, and I thought that what I experienced then and after would be of help to you, whether you are a patient or a prospective patient or part of a patient's circle of support. Before my own surgery I was particularly fortunate in having a few friends who had benefited from bypass surgery and a particularly close friend who was one of the pioneers in its development. Even with this system of support and information, most of what I experienced was a surprise—and sometimes a shock. Of course, I thought that the things I experienced were unique to me and was startled to learn that most of it was shared by other "veterans" I spoke to later. So why not tell you? Some of it, simple in itself, may save you worry and trouble. It has been said more than once that the main result of heart surgery is divorce. That's probably an exaggeration, but if we can circumvent a circuit overload or two we'll all be ahead of the game.

While this is not a scientific book, every effort has been made to confirm the truth of everything presented as *fact*. What is presented as *opinion*, however, is mine, and you are welcome to take it or leave it, as you like. It is simply offered to make life a little easier or healthier for you. One thing, though, about any advice I might offer: none of it will hurt you. Nothing, especially giving up smoking, will start you down some path of self-destruction.

Lest you feel you are alone, you are not. In 1993, the most recent year for which figures are available, 330,812 coronary artery bypass procedures were performed in the United States; 73 percent of them were on men and 49 percent on patients under age sixty-five. More importantly, after your surgery you will be one of millions of, in many cases, robust people given a new life by this extraordinary surgical procedure. The time will come when it will become obsolete, either because of the development of new techniques or the eradication of the plague that is heart disease, but today coronary artery bypass graft surgery is the most immediately effective relief for the symptoms of heart disease and the threat of heart attack. It truly offers a second chance.

There is a progression to one's encounter with this disease—from first chest pain to the actual surgery to noting the anniversaries of your operation—and for convenience I will use my own experience as a framework, particularly because it was almost the same as that of many other people I spoke with and is probably not unlike yours. I will stop along the way to offer you more detailed information on a few of the less obvious facts and procedures, some of which it's important for you to understand and some just to satisfy your curiosity. At the end of this book there is a glossary where you can find more detailed explanations and, I hope, clear definitions of all those terms you hear from your doctor or from others around you in the hospital. I'm sure to miss the one that confuses you, but I'll do my best not to.

Sudden confrontation with open heart surgery is shocking and traumatic, and seldom is there time to adjust to the idea before the reality begins. Take a minute out to consider the alternatives—continuing suffering, threat of heart attack, possible death—and take comfort in the fact that after the surgery is completed and your body has had a chance to recover, you will have the chance to live a new, healthier, possibly more fulfilling life. Think of this in navigational terms, as a mid-course correction, and choose the new path that's offered to you. However much you may have been blessed in your life, this is the single greatest opportunity in it. Grab it by the throat. Millions before you have.

Acknowledgments

First and foremost, I wish to thank George E. Green; he has been a good and supportive friend and he used his skills and experience to return my health to me. When he was asked how he could perform surgery on a personal friend, he replied in his quiet way, "I couldn't trust anyone else to do it." Most of all, it was his instincts about my symptoms which brought this all about. I am grateful to him beyond measure.

Arnold Phillips was my physician when this began, and he turned my case over to David Wolinsky, a cardiologist of great skill; David soon became a good friend. John Thomas Barnard took over when Dr. Wolinsky left New York, and he has taken excellent care of me when he has had the chance. I thank them with all my heart.

I certainly regret that I did not note the names of all those who cared for me during my stay in New York's St. Luke's Hospital around Thanksgiving of 1986. I would thank each of them personally, here, probably filling a page or more. They were kind and solicitous and profes-

sional, to a person, and I will never forget them. I also
wish to thank all those "veterans" who told me of their
own experiences and reactions; they were generous with
their time and feelings and enthusiasm.

The American Heart Association is a model of its kind.
Donna LaMarita and her successor, Shawna Prater, have
been of great help, responding to requests with prompt-
ness beyond the call of duty. Jennifer Rudin at the *Harvard
Health Letter* and Mark Abramowicz, M.D., of *The Medical
Letter on Drugs and Therapeutics*, were also generous with
work that had appeared in their own publications.

On a special occasion, my friend of many years, Sara
Hunter Hudson, organized a dinner party to introduce
my wife and me to friends of hers, the great scientist John
Vane and his wife, Daphne. Sir John and I turned out to
be "brothers under the skin," so to speak, fellow veterans
of coronary bypass surgery, and we spent a fine evening
becoming acquainted and comparing notes. He was enthusiastic about this project and has been so generous as
to say so publicly, for which I am very grateful.

I don't know which is worse: one's first encounter with
angina pectoris or losing an almost-finished book due to a
computer malfunction. I have experienced both and
would almost vote for the latter—perhaps because it is the
more recent shock. I was saved, and so was the book, by
Nat Jaeggli, who found a lot of chunks and bits and pieces
of text somewhere in cyberspace, and these king's horses
and king's men were able to put it back together again.
There may still be a brilliant phrase or sentence somewhere out there in the ether, but perhaps it will be the
seed for another book.

For very real reasons, but here *in pectore*, I wish to
thank our very dear friends Jeremy Gompertz, Robin Reif,
Amy Vance, and Barbara Worcester. Also, Joanna Pen-

nypacker was particularly kind to my wife and me at a very challenging time. We shall be aware of the humanity of each of them all our lives.

I do not see or speak with my son, Douglas R. Ewing, anywhere near as often as I would like. That is because he is in medical school, seeking the knowledge and skills that one day may allow him to perform the demanding surgery discussed in this book, or something equally challenging. My feeling is that he will become as fine a physician as he is a human being. Watching him grow and fulfill his promise has been, and remains, one of the great joys and deepest satisfactions of my life.

It remains to speak of two very special people. My wife, Birgitta, entered my life after my surgery and so missed the days of rich and riotous eating. Instead she has endured with me several years of hardship and anguish, not the least part of which was the death of our fathers within a brief period, with grace and faith and love way beyond reasonable expectation. She is an extraordinary person. Our son, Philip, is the most obvious sign of the second life made possible by bypass surgery.

And there is Nick Lyons. What a friend he has been, personally and professionally. He has guided me through the process of getting this book before your eyes and can truly be described as its "onlie begettor." He is as kind and personally generous a man as I have known, and his faith in me and this book has been sustaining. I thank him for his friendship and confidence from the bottom of my heart. Next summer we are going to fish together every day.

"Tell me where is fancie bred, or in the heart or in the head."

Shakespeare, *The Merchant of Venice* (II, 2, 64)

"Some persons hold, that there is a wisdom of the Head, and that there is a wisdom of the Heart."

Charles Dickens, *Hard Times*,
Book the Third, chapter 1

A Patient's Guide to Coronary Bypass Surgery and Its Aftermath

□ 1 □

The Surprise of a Lifetime— and Its Consequences

Late October–early November 1986: I was walking along in New York in the afternoon of one of those wonderful bright and clear fall days. All was right in the world— business was good, my son was distinguishing himself in school, and I felt a particular pride in him just then. It looked as though he might have some say as to where he would attend college, and I had watched his soccer team achieve a record of 14-0-2 in scheduled games and win its league championship and the first two games of the regional tournament (it would lose the championship game by a late goal, but never mind). Memories of a wonderful summer still lingered, friends were healthy and amusing and a joy to be with, and my head was beginning to be turned by an engaging woman I had recently met (by then I had been divorced for almost a decade). It was one of those rare times in life when one would change absolutely nothing.

I do not recall the mission that day but I shall never forget the event that would lead, years later, to this book. I quickened my pace for some forgotten reason and imme- diately became aware of a tightening in my chest, a severe pain in the left shoulder, a marked shortness of breath, and, most of all, very definite feelings of doom. I stopped dead in my tracks (if you'll excuse the expression) and in a matter of seconds it all went away. It was as though nothing had happened. Doubts lingered.

A few years earlier I had had a bout with bursitis, that painful inflammation of the shoulder joint, and two or three days before the incident in the street I had suspected the onset of a chest cold. Surely these singly or in combination were to blame. Besides, I was very busy just then and certainly did not have time for some kind of health problem, for heaven's sake.

An intensified repetition of these symptoms a day or two later—on a Sunday morning, I well remember, and this time it was *really* frightening—led me to call a doctor friend who had diagnosed and miraculously "cured" my bursitis several years before. Was this a heart attack? I wondered. He made time in his very busy schedule to see me the next day, and a brief physical examination and a few questions was all he needed to dismiss the possibility of bursitis or anything like it. "Better call Arnie Phillips," Bill said, referring to the family doctor to whom he had introduced my son and me. "Now would be a good time." Dr. Phillips *told* me—it was decidedly not a suggestion— to meet him at the hospital as soon as I could get there. No more than a few minutes were required after my arrival to attach me to the electrocardiogram, or EKG, machine. Soon from its side spewed the paper tape on which my future could be read. It did not take Dr. Phillips and his colleague long to identify the source of the discomfort: coronary heart disease, the country's number one killer, and its dramatic and specific symptom, angina pectoris, the chest pain I had experienced. I was stunned. I was forty-three years old.

There is coincidence and there is luck. Then way

beyond both there is extraordinary good fortune. Mine was in the form of a friend, someone for whom I had great affection and trust; when we were together we discussed just about everything except his business and my health. He is a heart surgeon (in many ways, *the* heart surgeon) and my health was, all of a sudden, in jeopardy. I called him that evening and our conversation was more focused than usual. I was to travel to Albany—I then lived in New York City, so it was not too long a journey—to undergo coronary angiography. Albany because the master of this skill—almost an art, really—practiced there: Dr. Julio Sosa. My doctor friend explained that these pictures of the heart and its arteries were the only *real* way to determine if there was coronary artery disease, and how extensive it might be. As for me, I was too numb to protest this journey.

The train to Albany arrived early if I remember correctly—why couldn't it have been late just this once?—and I spent most of the afternoon in the hospital for the preliminary physical examination and X rays. This was followed by a solitary dinner and an early night at a nearby hotel, since I was to report back to the hospital (without breakfast!) at something like 7 A.M. I wish I could say I was looking forward to the next day, but this is not a work of fiction.

Coronary angiography is carried out under the most strict surgical conditions so as to avoid infection, but there were not as many delays at the hospital as I would have liked. The procedure is basically very simple although the technology involved is complex, and before I knew it the catheter had been inserted into the brachial artery in my right arm (an alternative route starts in the groin and uses the femoral artery), threaded down into my chest, and carefully guided into my left coronary artery, the most important of the heart's sources of blood since it supplies the pump that sends fresh blood out to the rest of the body. I could actually *see* that artery and the rest of *my own* heart on the television monitor. It's a cliché, I know, but it was unbelievable. Dr. Sosa's film showed a strong, intact heart muscle but serious blockage—technically 98 percent stenosis—in the main one or left anterior descending, and lesser, but still serious disease in the two other arteries. There was a good chance I would have a heart attack in the not-too-distant future and likely that it would be a serious one—perhaps fatal! On the other hand, I was an ideal candidate for Coronary Artery Bypass Graft surgery: relatively young, otherwise healthy, with an undamaged heart muscle. My insurance was paid up and, what was most important to me, my son was mature and old enough to go the rest of the way on his own, should that become necessary. Dr. Sosa telephoned my friend, and soon-to-be surgeon, George Green, and then broke the news to me: I needed quadruple bypass surgery as soon as possible, without its being an emergency (heart surgery seldom is). Thanksgiving was a few weeks away and the day before it seemed like a good day to perform the surgery. This would give me some time to get organized.

I suppose I have felt more alone before, but I sure don't know when. I have not since. The train ride home, along a darkening Hudson River in the late afternoon of a gloomy November day, is useful to think back on when events seem to be other than they should be.

What had I done to put myself in this position? Should I have heeded those warnings on cigarette packages and stopped smoking? Should I have paid attention to my "cholesterol"—whatever that was? I had vague memories of a doctor telling me to keep an eye on it some years before. Should I not have stopped exercising so long ago? Did I drink too much? Was I going to die soon? What had I done—or not done—to deserve this? These and many other questions clamored for attention.

And I had so many things to do! As soon as I was home I sat down to list them. I soon abandoned this for fear of spending my remaining time making lists and not doing what needed to be done. First of all, of course, I had to tell my son and then my close friends (of which I have, I am glad to say, a good number). Then business arrangements and all the other matters we—or at least I—are so skilled at avoiding when they are not pressing. The last days before surgery were a blur, but I somehow managed to accomplish all that I *needed* to do, including telling the woman I was beginning to date that no, I could not go to a party with her the next weekend, much as I would like to, because I was having open heart surgery next Wednesday. She nearly fell off her chair.

The toughest part, of course, was informing my son, who at seventeen had his feet pretty firmly on the ground and was focused on his application for early admission to college. I *think* he was pretty shaken, but do you know anyone that age who would show it? He was not reduced to tears, but he was pretty quiet for some time.

It was certainly a strange sensation leaving the busy world of the well to enter the world of a large metropolitan hospital, especially on a bright and sunny morning when I felt no kinship to those not in control of their own destinies. My own symptoms seemed far away. Maybe the last tests before surgery would indicate an unexpected improvement! But in any event, I was obliged to be at the hospital in time to be admitted before the special class they give to the next day's heart surgery patients.

I did not need much in the hospital and you won't

either: pajamas or a nightshirt, a robe, slippers, a toilet kit, a book or two, and I found a few photographs from happier times to be most welcome. It is wise to remember that you will be away from your room for the few days you spend in the recovery room, so don't take along anything valuable—and you certainly won't be needing a watch. You will be glad that you brought a change of comfortable street clothes on the first day you begin to feel human again and the days that follow.

The admissions procedures make you realize who *really* runs the hospital, and I was just barely in time for the last orientation class. It was brief. I won't try to repeat what I was told then because I have absolutely no memory of it. There is only one thing you have to know before your surgery, however, and that is that the first thing you will probably be aware of when you wake up is someone beating you. No, your family and friends are not taking advantage of your unconscious state to settle accounts: mucus collects in the lungs during surgery and it is important to loosen it and cough it up before it can develop into pneumonia. So a nurse will pound on your back just when you want to be left alone. You will not even have the will to resent it.

Preoperative care lacks the drama and intensity of what will follow—in fact it seems pretty casual—but in its own way it is every bit as important. You will have been given instructions whether or not to continue the medications you have been taking, and it would be a good idea to take a few minutes just to list them, their dosage and frequency, *before* you go to the hospital, because it is very important that you not forget anything. This even includes aspirin, and is particularly true for medicines you take for conditions *other than* your heart disease, like allergies.

At least one, and possibly more, complete physical examination awaits you, and there will be many questions from several people about your medical history. If this seems unrelated to your heart disease it is not: your body will soon be undergoing an enormous number of physical and chemical changes and continuous monitoring and adjusting will be necessary; what is normal for *you*, not for the textbook ideal, must be determined so that it can be used as a guide. Similarly, such factors as your blood clotting speed, say, or your blood sugar level or sensitivity to certain kinds of drugs are essential for the doctors to know. The complete physical examination is necessary to make sure that you don't have a problem that would complicate the surgery or suggest its postponement. A hitherto undiscovered infection in a seemingly unrelated part of the body, for instance, could easily put the success of the surgery, and your life, in jeopardy. You will probably also be given an antibiotic as a precaution against any unknown infection or minute disturbance that might occur tomorrow.

After class you will go to your room for what should be the longest, but will probably be the shortest, afternoon of your life. Whatever blood tests you might have had recently will be repeated, with more thrown in for good measure; a urine sample will be sought and not easily produced; the anesthesiologist will visit you to discuss your general health and any allergies you might have. *Your answers are extremely important!* Just as the surgeon has to tailor the surgery to you and your unique needs, the doctor who will keep you unconscious during the operation needs to plan what will work best for you: the days of an ether-soaked mask clamped over the face are long gone. Think before you reply. Other visitors will probably include: a surgical resident or two (or three or four) to ask a lot of questions about your medical history; someone to take yet another electrocardiogram, that painless procedure with all the cups or small plates and profusion of wires that records your heart's electric impulses; an orderly or operating room technician to shave or clip the hair on your chest, a mildly unpleasant but necessary procedure; your cardiologist and/or family physician, or the one who has been assigned to you; your surgeon, whom you may not have met before (don't be offended if he or she is abrupt; where you want undivided attention is *tomorrow*, and you'll get it); the hospital chaplain or your own priest or clergyperson or rabbi; the dietician; an X-ray technician or two; your floor nurse, with questions or medication. In other words, if I were you I would not put off an important chore until this afternoon. Leave it open.

I had felt varying degrees of anxiety almost continuously since those first chest pains, but strangely enough my last evening before the operation was anxiety-free. Knowing I was under highly competent care is one reason, of course, and so is its corollary, knowing I would have no decisions or even choices to make for a while. But there is another, less easily discussed, matter, too, and it is called letting go. As adults we at least like to think we have a fair degree of control over our own lives, and as parents we have had to exercise almost absolute control over the lives of others. Indeed, control of one sort or another is a major matter in most adult lives and leaving it behind, even if only temporarily, can be difficult. Letting go is simply putting your own life in God's hands. It is not a reduced will to live—far from it!—but it is an acceptance that you might not live and realizing that that is okay, too. Once you have let go, of course, there is no fear, for fear is the threat of harm. To put it as simply as possible, letting go is *knowing*, not just thinking or hoping, that no harm can befall you. The conclusion I came to was that Death had an extremely effective P.R. agent and that there was much less there than met the eye. But there were still lots of fish—in salt water and fresh—to catch before that became an issue!

An early dinner will be followed by a brief but quiet evening. After a meal of which I have no memory—this can unfortunately be said of most hospital meals, but never mind—I went into the solarium or lounge or whatever they called it to smoke a cigarette. My surgeon friend dropped by to see me on his way home and asked if I was enjoying my smoke. Yes, of course, I replied. "Good, I hope so. It will be your last." And so it was.

The two visitors I had that evening stand out in memory: my lady friend brought a gift of good cheer and optimism and left with laughter still in the air; the lady who was my clergyman (if that construction isn't sexist) and also my pastor brought me reassurance and reaffirmation of faith, yes, but most importantly, love. I went to bed fairly early, planning to read for a while and not expecting to get much sleep. Wrong. The sedative I had been given did its work quickly.

THE DAY, November 26, 1986, dawned like most other days in my life—without my observing it. I was awakened soon enough for that last question or test, and before I knew it the transportation team from the operating room was knocking on my door. I had been given another medication of some sort and details of my ride down hospital corridors are not clear, nor are they important. If you are the day's first patient—a given operating room normally accommodates two patients each day—you will probably go right into the room where you will spend the next five or six hours; if not, you may wait briefly in the

corridor or "parking lot," convinced, and perhaps praying, that you have been forgotten and can sneak quietly
away. You haven't been and you can't. The wait will seem
forever and not long enough. In any event, even the
medication you've been given won't prevent those last
thoughts: did I remember to do such and such? Will my
son (or daughter or wife or whatever) be okay? I was much
comforted knowing my friends Vivien and Bill Clark were
looking after my son. Bill was the physician on whom I
was able to blame my presence here and Bill would be able
to answer, indeed anticipate, my son's questions; Vivien,
his wife, was—and is—one of those rare take-charge
people in whose hands you know *anything* is safe. She
was, and is, one of my oldest and closest friends. Was I
ever thankful for them!

Because you will undergo a surgical procedure not
unlike mine, I am now going to offer you a brief and
accurate description of it. If you are squeamish, you may
not wish to read it just now, so skip it and return to it
when you're of a mind to. Unlike almost everything else
about your disease, there's nothing here you *must* know,
but some knowledge of the rigors of the surgery may
induce you to do what is necessary to avoid another such
operation. What *is* important to know, though, is that you
will have *no* awareness or memory of what goes on during
surgery. That's the one part that is entirely in the hands of
the surgeon and his (or her) team—and it *is* a team, in
every way, including size. So we'll just let them get on
with their business.

□ 2 □

The Main Event

Preparations for surgery begin with an injection well before your journey to the operating room. This medication has four purposes: drying of internal fluids, reduction of anxiety, and promotion of both drowsiness and amnesia. None of the effects will be dramatic and you would probably not be aware of them had you not been informed.

All the information about your medical history and personal foibles that you provided in those many interviews has been combined with the results of laboratory tests to construct a program of anesthesia specifically for you. Advances in this field of medicine have been as extensive and dramatic as those in others but are not publicized, basically because of lack of relevance to everyday life. The goals are to keep you free of pain, unaware of what is taking place, free of memory of the trauma your body is experiencing, but not so deeply unconscious that your body is unable to function normally—indeed strongly!—and respond to the many demands and tests that will be asked of it. While you are asleep, it is to be hoped blissfully, your body will be experiencing more challenges than ever before.

The physician in charge of the anesthesia is in fact a highly trained specialist called an anesthesiologist; his (or her) responsibilities during surgery extend far beyond making sure you don't wake up at the wrong time. Every procedure your body endures, every medication administered, will produce a reaction, and the anesthesiologist must adjust and "fine tune" continuously. He receives the information from all the various monitors and probes and keeps constant watch on the body's chemistry. He supervises the perfusionist, whom we will meet soon, and is generally in charge of you and your well-being so that the surgeon can concentrate on his work. The anesthesiologist or his assistant will also escort you to the coronary care unit to make sure your breathing is normal and your monitors are all functioning properly. But don't expect to be able to thank him then.

Before you move to the operating room table from the rolling stretcher, called a gurney, electrodes from the electrocardiogram monitor will be attached to your back. This machine will be running constantly during the procedure and will immediately alert the surgeon of any sudden or unexpected changes in normal heart patterns. After a small injection of local anesthetic, the first IV or intravenous tube will be inserted into a vein in your wrist or arm; this will be used to administer anesthesia and to maintain normal body moisture and nutrition by way of the IV drip; many of the medications you will need will also use this conduit. As you begin to lose consciousness, other catheters will be put in place, to maintain your body's stability and monitor its functions: a Foley, or urinary, catheter will be put in the bladder to prevent unsanitary conditions, but more importantly to monitor the functioning of the kidneys, those organs so crucial to your health. One, called a central line, will be threaded down either the jugular vein in the neck or the subclavian vein near the collarbone, into the vena cava, the large vein next to the heart, to deliver medication directly to the heart if necessary. A radial artery catheter will measure oxygen levels and pressure in the arteries, and a particularly elegant detector called a Swan-Ganz catheter will be inserted through an incision in a vein in the neck and guided into the right heart, through the right ventricle and the pulmonic valve into the pulmonary artery and lung. This will monitor temperature, pulmonary artery blood pressure, heart function, and it is also able to deliver medication directly to the heart. When the surgery is completed, two rubber tubes will be inserted in the pericardium and "externalized"—drawn outside through a hole on either side of the chest just a few inches below the nipple; these tubes will drain the cavity of excess fluid, most notably blood that did not benefit from the recoagulation medication administered at the end of the surgery. The tubes will be removed a day or so after surgery and the only memory they will leave behind will be two little scars.

After you have lost consciousness, an endotracheal tube will be placed in your windpipe so that a respirator can assume control of your breathing; a nasogastric tube will be placed through the nose to the stomach so that fluids there can be removed. A drug called heparin will be administered to "thin" the blood and prevent clotting. Simultaneously, your chest will be swabbed with a strong antiseptic solution to prevent contamination.

With the catheters and other tubes in place, an assisting surgeon will make an incision somewhere in your leg to remove or "harvest" several eight-inch lengths of saphenous vein: one to be be used for each planned vein bypass and one kept in reserve even when only arterial grafts are planned. The minor discomfort this will leave is likely to be what you notice most during the early stages of recovery.

At about the same time the chief surgeon or his assistant (also a highly trained and experienced cardiovascular surgeon) will begin the operation with an incision precisely down the middle of your chest, from just below the collarbone to about three inches below the bottom of the rib cage. After the small amount of bleeding is attended to, a very sharp oscillating saw is used to divide the sternum, the chest bone, along the same straight line of the incision. This approach, from the front, is called a median sternotomy. A chest spreader is then inserted so that the chest can be kept open. Great care is taken to insure even and comfortable healing.

Assuming the internal thoracic arteries, or ITAs, are to be used, the sternum is elevated on one side and held up with a piece of hardware called a self-retaining sternal retractor. This allows the surgeon to gently separate the artery from the chest wall and clamp it off. If both sides are to be used this procedure is repeated on the other side, and both arteries are then trimmed and tidied in preparation for use. Next the pericardium, the sac of tissue that protects the heart, is cut open to expose the heart itself. Inspection will reveal any damage to the heart muscle caused by heart attacks, and large arterial occlusions should be visible. The observations and plans made on the basis of angiograms and other evidence will also be confirmed by on-site inspection.

The Heart-Lung Machine

It is now time for the extraordinary and indispensable device (more formally called a cardiopulmonary bypass machine) that allows the heart to be stopped, repaired, and started again, none the worse for its time in the shop. A moving, beating heart, of course, would make the very delicate surgery that is soon to come impossible to perform. The technician who operates this machine is called a perfusionist.

More heparin is administered to further insure against clotting and an incision is made in the right atrium; after clamping, a plastic tube is inserted and tied in place. This will take the "used" blood from the heart to the machine. A similar tube is inserted into the aorta and secured there, to take "fresh" blood from the machine back to the body just as if it had come from the lungs and heart. The machine cleans the blood of waste and impurities, oxygenates it, and pumps it back with force comparable to that of the heart.

The heart needs less oxygen and is better preserved if its temperature is reduced considerably, and this is done in three ways: the heart itself is flushed with a cold saline solution; the blood in the machine is cooled by surrounding the tubes carrying it with ice; and a cold potassium solution called cardioplegia solution is injected directly into the heart, which also stops the heart's electrical activity. With careful monitoring and judicious repeated use of the cardioplegia solution, preservation of the heart's tissues is insured for up to six hours.

After all attachments are checked carefully, the clamps are removed and the machine started. There is not even a millisecond's gap in the normal functioning of *all* the organs in the body except the heart and lungs, which are taking their first "breather" in your life.

Depending on the number, extent, and location of the occlusions in your arteries, your surgeon's skills and preferences, and your own physical resources, your surgeon will have planned your bypass grafts from among these choices:

1. *The artery graft*. The internal thoracic artery, or ITA,

formerly known as the internal mammary artery, branches off the subclavian artery approximately at the collarbone and descends the inner chest wall to about the space between the sixth and seventh ribs, where it branches in two. In this method the artery is separated from the chest wall (it lies under a thin layer of muscle tissue), clamped twice just above the bifurcation, and the bottom half tied off. The free end is then passed through a small hole in the pericardium and grafted to the coronary artery between the blockage and the heart muscle. This is called a pedicle graft, and statistics have shown it to be the most reliable and long-lived, for demonstrable reasons. If arteries from both sides of the chest are used we speak of bilateral grafts.

2. *The vein graft.* One end of a length of vein, usually from the saphenous vein in the leg, is grafted to the coronary artery between the blockage and the heart muscle and the other is grafted into the aorta, where fresh blood goes immediately after leaving the heart. This is called a free graft.

3. *The hybrid.* A free graft as described above, but using a length of artery instead of vein.

There is a further variation within these categories: if multiple grafts are made with a single length of vein or artery, it is said to be sequential.

There has also been success using two other arteries for pedicle grafts: the right gastroepiploic, which runs from right to left along the great curvature of the stomach, and the inferior epigastric, which arises from the external iliac artery just above the urinary bladder and ascends in the front of the abdomen. Use of these arteries began fairly recently, so there are no long-term reports of success as yet, but the inferior epigastric artery would seem to offer the most promise. These arteries would be used not as alternatives to the traditional choices but only when ITA and saphenous vein grafts are not feasible.

You can't imagine how small the coronary arteries and other vessels are until you actually see them, and the skill required to accomplish this suturing (otherwise the operation is quite simple *in principle*) is just amazing to watch. The success of the operation—*your future*—depends on the surgeon's skills and experience: precise sewing here means no leakage and sufficient blood flow or patency.

Although surgeons in other fields (notably eye and brain surgeons) have taken to the surgical microscope like the proverbial duck to water, cardiovascular surgeons have been slow to adapt to it, stating a preference for a small magnifying loupe. I can't explain why this is true, but it is. It is important to note that surgeons who have learned to use the microscope and have become comfortable with it in the laboratory recommend its use strongly and speak of very convincing results with it. To quote Eugene Flamm, a world-famous neurosurgeon whose specialty is the brain's vascular system, "The greatest recent advance has come about with our ability to see what we're doing. That sounds a little facetious. But using the microscope in the operating room has brought about incredible changes about what can be done surgically. Some people advocated it early on and one person [Dr. M. Gazi Yasargil of Zurich] went a long way in demanding that everyone use it."

I think there is little doubt that in time all such surgery will use this superb aid.

When the grafts are completed, they are tested and any needed adjustments made; once all is satisfactory the aortic clamp is removed and the blood gradually warmed. This is usually enough to prompt the heart to start beating again, but if not, a small electric shock called cardioversion will give it the necessary boost. Once the heart is beating, the machine is stopped, the tubes are removed from the aorta and right atrium, and the operation goes into reverse: the pericardium is closed, the two drainage tubes externalized, the chest spreader loosened and removed, and the ribs carefully matched and sewn together with stainless steel wire. The skin is sutured, the wound cleaned and bandaged, and it's all over. On the several occasions I have observed this, the mood of satisfaction, pride, and relief in the operating room was palpable. Everyone had made a significant contribution to giving a very sick, indeed dying, person a second chance at life. A sick person had been made well. As many times as these people do this—and they often do it several times a day—the very special nature of this work is not lost on them.

❑ 3 ❑

The Prince in a Kingdom

The heart, ready furnished with its proper organ of motion . . . existed before the body. The first to be formed, nature willed that it should afterwards fashion, nourish, preserve the entire animal, as its work and dwelling place: and as the prince in a kingdom. . . .

William Harvey, . . . de motu cordis . . . , 1628

While, figuratively speaking, you are occupied in the operating room, let's take some time to explain how you came to be where you are. It will be several days before you are consistently aware of what is going on around you, and it should be worthwhile to have this information, or at least know where to look for it. If you are at all like I was, you have a pretty good idea of what this is all about but are (also like I was) misinformed.

Now that we finally have a few minutes to sit down and reflect on it all, what you are going through is close to overwhelming. Here you are, right in the middle of your adult life: you have probably managed to get your life on track—marriage doing fine, kids through school or close to it, job okay—perhaps not quite all that you had hoped for but certainly not as bad as it could be. You very likely have survived some tough obstacles along the way. Retirement, while perhaps still in the future, intrudes into your thoughts from time to time. Now this! If you haven't had a heart attack, you certainly have had a bad scare from that chest pain and there is always the threat of heart attack. Before you even knew what was happening you were told to report to the hospital for open heart surgery. And you're not even sick! It's the most frightening thing that's ever happened to you and things couldn't be any worse. Right?

Wrong. You probably don't know how lucky you are, and you'll go through some real discomfort before you do. But it really is only discomfort; there's very little pain involved and what there is is altogether bearable. When the surgery and recuperation are all over, you'll think that despite the brusqueness, your surgeon is the greatest person on earth (in fact he or she probably is) and you are the luckiest. You are. I am, too.

When you were a child there was probably someone you knew—as often as not a relative—who was functionally an invalid. He or she stayed at home most of the time, went out seldom, always walked very slowly, looked as pale as could be, and spoke slowly and without animation. When you asked what was wrong, the reply was "heart condition," spoken in hushed tones. As far as you were concerned such people were the living dead. There were hundreds of thousands of them across the country.

Do you recall how many people in their late fifties or early sixties used to keel over suddenly and either die or become an invalid for their few remaining years? That's where you were headed, and up until very recently there was nothing that anyone could have done about it. What you are about to have, Coronary Artery Bypass Graft surgery—and yes, inevitably, the medical jargon is "cabbage"—was dreamed about and planned and hoped for and prayed for by many people for many years, but not successfully performed until 1967! (Actually, there was a single, isolated, successful bypass performed in 1964, but it went unreported—one of the most bizarre nonevents in medical history. This strange tale is recounted briefly in the appendix). That was less than thirty years ago. The story of this development, by the way, is a fascinating one and is told later on; it includes names that would include at least half my pantheon of twentieth-century medical heroes: Beck, Favaloro, Forssmann, Gibbon, Green, Sones, Vineberg; you probably don't recognize the names, but because of their work hundreds of thousands, no, millions, of lives—especially yours and mine!—either have been saved or, even more important, *made livable*. So before we proceed, let's tip our hats to these our heroes.

The simple fact is that less than thirty years ago you might well have died or become an invalid, and now you will undergo some anxiety, a lot of inconvenience, and a fair amount of discomfort, and before long you will be *much healthier than you are now*. You will have a chance to undo the damage you have been doing to yourself all these years, by changing your diet, exercising, and QUIT-TING SMOKING, and you'll now have an excellent chance of actually seeing those grandchildren as they grow into young adults, and enjoying those retirement years you and your spouse had planned, and whatever else you had hoped for in the future. Because there *will* be a future.

But before we get too involved in the future, let's take a look at the present and at the part of the past that brought us here. It's not as much of a detour as you might think, because in it lies the explanation of why you are where you are. I'll try not to be too technical. I am not a scientist, but since I have heart disease, I felt compelled to understand it and its effects. It is not particularly complicated. If you are at all like me, you were taken by surprise and are in a state of shock. As the doctor was patiently explaining what heart disease was and why you needed surgery, you were thinking, How much work will I miss? Will my insurance cover all of the cost? How can I pay for it? Do I have to stop smoking? The focus of my attention was whether or not I would be allowed to travel to attend a friend's fiftieth birthday party (I was and I did). All of this, of course, is our mind's not-so-subtle way of diverting our attention from the very frightening fact that we have a potentially catastrophic illness, and if we don't watch out we're going to be in big trouble.

To begin with and just to confuse the issue, heart disease is not. The term *heart disease* evokes the image of a heart-shaped mass of disease and infection, but in fact, your heart itself is likely to be quite healthy. Heart disease is more accurately called coronary heart disease, and it is the symptoms and features of coronary artery disease. The coronary arteries that supply the heart with blood are affected, not the heart itself. The disease in the arteries is more accurately called atherosclerosis and is occasionally referred to as "hardening of the arteries."

The heart itself is a muscle and is more specifically called the myocardium; it is subdivided into four compartments (the right and left atria and the right and left ventricles), and these in turn have four valves (the tricuspid and mitral are between the atria and the ventricles; the pulmonic is between the right ventricle and the pulmonary artery; and the aortic is at the mouth of the aorta, at the top of the left ventricle). The function of the heart is to pump used—that is to say, oxygen-poor—blood into the lungs to get resupplied with oxygen, and oxygen-enriched blood from the lungs back to the body. The "new" blood goes out in arteries and "used" blood returns in veins, and these are called collectively blood vessels. All of this together is called the circulatory system, and it extends to every part of the body, with its very smallest branches called capillaries. Disease of any of these blood vessels is called vascular disease.

In the upper wall of the right atrium near the entry of the vena cava is a microscopic area of specialized heart muscle known as the sinoatrial or SA node. This is Action Central—the "pacemaker" that sends electrical signals to control the heartbeat. Of particular importance is its signal to the atrioventricular node, a mass of modified heart muscle in the lower middle part of the right atrium; this, called the AV node, controls the contraction of the atrium and sends along the signal to the ventricles by way of the atrioventricular bundle. The heart, like much else in the world, is run by electrical signals.

Just for fun, let's trace the round trip of a single drop of blood as it takes oxygen to the body's tissues and picks up carbon dioxide and other waste gases for excretion. Beginning in the left ventricle, the force of the contracting heart muscle pushes the blood through the aortic valve into the aorta and down a series of progressively smaller arteries and finally arterioles; thence into capillaries, venules, and progressively larger veins into either the superior (from the upper part of the body) or inferior (from the lower part of the body) vena cava into the right atrium, thence through the tricuspid valve into the right ventricle, through the pulmonic valve and pulmonic artery into the lungs, where the blood leaves behind the carbon dioxide and other waste gases and acquires oxygen, thereby becoming bright red again. From the lungs, it flows through one of the four pulmonary veins into the left atrium, through the mitral valve into the left ventricle, where the journey began.

Probably the most important of all of the vessels are the ones closest to home, those that service the heart itself. You would think that with all the blood moving around inside it the heart would just help itself to what was there, like a diner at the buffet table, but that is not the way it works. The first blood vessels to branch from the aorta are the two coronary arteries, so named from the Latin word *corona*, which means crown. It only requires a little stretch of the imagination to picture them on top of the heart and branching down, like a wax crown drooping in the heat.

The two coronary arteries are the left and the right. The left, or left main, is the larger and more important since it supplies the left ventricle (which pumps blood to the body) with fresh blood. An inch or so from the aorta, this artery sends off a branch which becomes the left circumflex (LCA) and this curves around the heart; the main continues as the left anterior descending (LAD). The right coronary artery (RCA) descends and provides blood to the right side of the heart. As both arteries descend and get farther from the aorta they divide into smaller and smaller branches, providing a network of blood supply looking not unlike a tree's root system.

There are about ten pints of blood in the body and two and a half ounces of it are pushed out with each beat of the heart (a thousand gallons every twenty-four hours!). When the body is at rest, the trip we just took requires about a minute, but with moderate exercise that can increase to four times a minute. The network of blood vessels if stretched out would be about sixty thousand miles—two and a half times around the world.

Without our telling it to, the heart beats regularly, without *ever* taking a rest, from before birth to (sometimes) after death, an average of more than 50 times a minute; 3,000 times an hour; 72,000 times a day; 2 million times a month; 24 million times a year—more than 2 *billion* times in the average seventy-two-year life-span. When you stop to think about it—and this is a good time to do just that—that's a really astonishing feat. The heart can withstand a great deal of abuse—dead tissue, damaged valves, infection, shock—and still go on beating as long as it is fed continuously with blood. When the supply stops, the heart literally starves to death, and "death" occurs very quickly. Of course when our hearts die, we do, too.

The coronary arteries can be compared to water pipes, and like pipes they may get clogged. Just as impurities in water build up on the interior of a pipe, obstructions can accumulate in the coronary arteries. These obstructions are called atheromas, or plaques, and are composed of a waxy substance called cholesterol, other fats called triglycerides, and/or scar tissue. As this build-up hardens, a condition called atherosclerosis, the flow of blood past the blockage decreases. Often a clot, or thrombus, will form, further increasing the danger. When the blood supply becomes too low or too slow, several things can happen: angina pectoris, the strongest possible warning of trouble and the heart's cry for more blood; a myocardial infarction (or M.I. in medical slang, not to be confused with MCI, which wants to be your long distance telephone company), commonly known as a heart attack, which means that some heart tissue has actually died of malnutrition; and death.

Detection and Diagnosis

Detection and diagnosis of coronary disease is complex, since chest pain and shortness of breath are the principal symptoms and these can have other sources: a cold or other respiratory affliction, lung disease, allergies, a strained muscle, even indigestion, not to mention the fact that we can easily persuade ourselves that our symptoms *do* have other sources. Angina pectoris, literally "strangulation of the chest," is a dramatic indication of trouble. Shortness of breath, tightness or other pain or discomfort in various places in the chest, pain in the neck or jaw or even teeth, strange feelings or heaviness in either or both arms, a kind of indigestion never felt before are all possible symptoms. It has probably never been described better than by William Heberden, the English physician who in 1722 first used the term and wrote: "They who are afflicted with it are seized while they are walking...with a painful and most disagreeable sensation in the breast, which seems as if it would extinguish life, if it were to increase or continue; but the moment they stand still, all this uneasiness vanishes."

Two symptoms are almost invariably present: the sense that the heart is literally being squeezed, and feelings of doom, which diminish in time. A very strong indication of coronary artery involvement is the disappearance of symptoms with brief rest. When the discomfort appears and disappears virtually on command with exertion or emotional stress, the condition is called stable angina; when it is less predictable, unstable angina. Occasionally it is totally unpredictable, occurring at rest as well as during exertion and that condition is called Prinzmetal angina, after the man who first described it. There is also a rather mysterious condition called coronary spasm, which is a sudden contraction in a segment of the coronary artery, obstructing the flow of blood to the heart muscle, the same as if by blockage. Of course there is increased danger if the artery is already blocked, a narrowing of an already narrow passage. This phenomenon is most frequently associated with emotional stress.

Several diagnostic procedures help to confirm and define the extent of the disease. A careful history taken by a skilled diagnostician is an important start and may well reveal more than a physical examination or an X ray, although both of these are necessary since an altogether different source of the discomfort might be discovered. A resting electrocardiogram (EKG), that painless procedure with all the wires attached to you, *might* show something, but then again might not; its more complex—and demanding—extension, the exercise EKG, or stress test, is more likely to produce useful information. With only the chest leads in place, the patient walks on a treadmill; as the speed and angle are increased, physical stress is induced to test the limit of the blood supply to the heart. Blood pressure and heart rate are monitored and the test is stopped if these exceed expectation based on predetermined levels of a normal range of tolerance based on physical condition, known history, and age. Of course it is also stopped if unexpected chest pain develops.

The purpose of the test is to measure tolerance for exercise and to see if angina is induced. If the test is tolerated, the results are said to be "negative"; if it is demonstrated that the heart is not receiving an adequate supply of blood, the results are "positive," thus making it that kind of test you would yearn to fail.

If a heart attack is suspected to have occurred, or as a post-surgical determination of the surgery's effectiveness, a similar test is used. At the peak of exercise a radioisotope of the element thallium (actually thallium-201) is injected in the arm, and after a while the heart is X-rayed. Any areas of the heart *not* reached by the thallium show up as "cold" spots and indicate damage to that part of the heart muscle. Similar tests are performed with the radioactive tracers sestamibi and teboroxime.

The exercise stress test indicates the *presence* of the disease but not the *extent*, which brings us to the ultimate diagnostic technique, one of the crowning glories of modern medicine: coronary angiography.

In this procedure, which is done in a hospital, a narrow, flexible tube called a catheter is inserted into a blood vessel in either the arm or the groin and carefully guided toward the heart. Once there, it is manipulated into the left or main coronary artery, all of which is carefully observed through a fluoroscope. Dye is released and X-ray movies (cineangiography) taken. These movies record the condition of the arteries on the left side of the heart and reveal the degree of blockage or occlusion, if any. Equally important, they show the *location* of the obstructions—essential information for therapeutic strategy. A fairly simple manipulation of the catheter allows access to the right side of the heart, but this is seldom necessary.

There is one thing I will add here and can do so only because this is not a scientific work. There is *no* evidence to support this association, not even common sense— particularly not common sense! But many of the people with heart disease, I among them, have a small fold in the lower earlobe, and I would suspect that many experienced cardiologists might secretly place much weight on this factor (but don't ask!). When the mapping of the human gene is completed many years from now, it will not surprise me to see verification of this association. I believe other such apparently unrelated phenomena are known. I offer no explanations other than that we still have a lot to learn about the human body. Just think how much we have learned in the past thirty years!

Treatment

With the information provided by these tests, and taking into consideration anything else that is relevant, such as the age and general health of the patient, doctor and patient and the patient's family can now set about choosing an appropriate course of treatment, since these blockages must either be cleared out or circumvented or there will be hell to pay. This treatment can take several different forms, and each of them has its advantages and disadvantages.

1. *Diet*. Obviously the most "natural" and one of the two noninvasive methods. Since cholesterol is building up, we eliminate sources of it from the diet and add food with cholesterol-reducing properties. Then we wait and hope for the best.

The best thing about this method is that it is painless and we don't have the trauma of surgery, with its possible side effects. The worst thing is that it is difficult to monitor its efficacy or progress. Combined with exercise and stress reduction, a radical diet has been shown to work. The possibility of a heart attack, however, is still very real.

2. *Drug therapy*. A course of medication is prescribed by your cardiologist. This could include drugs which reduce cholesterol levels in your blood; slow and regulate your heartbeat; lower your blood pressure; prevent constriction of the coronary arteries; widen arteries

throughout the body; and any combination of these. Once again, we have not opened up the body and subjected it to the indignities of surgery and once again, progress cannot be easily monitored. And in addition to the continuing threat of a heart attack, we have added the unknown factor of possible adverse reaction to the drugs.

3. *Angioplasty.* The procedure described above as angiography is repeated, but this time the catheter is equipped with a tiny inflatable device, so the technique is also called balloon angioplasty, or more technically percutaneous transluminal coronary angioplasty or PTCA. The balloon is guided into position above or between the blockage and inflated. This presses down the plaque and the flow of blood is immediately improved. The patient spends a few hours in supervised recovery—really more to recover from the drugs used to induce relaxation than for the trauma of the procedure—and returns home, probably little the worse for wear. (There is a slight risk involved, however: the mortality rate is about 0.1 percent, or one in a thousand.)

At first glance this would seem to be the treatment of choice: maximum reduction of blockage in minimum time with minimum wear and tear. What more could one ask for, save a magic pill? Unfortunately, there is more to it than this.

First of all, the procedure should be used only when the blockage is high in the coronary arteries and easily accessible (the catheter is introduced from above). Second, the atheroma should be single, not a series, that is to say the disease must not be diffuse. Third, the very act of inducing a catheter into the left coronary artery, where the disease is likely to be, can itself produce a heart attack, the very event we're trying to prevent. Fourth, the material from the blockage dislodged by the catheter may now be moving around in the bloodstream. It might dissolve or be filtered out somewhere, but it might also drop anchor and settle down and cause infection, abscess, or even a hemorrhage. Fifth, the very procedure of crushing the plaque into the wall of the artery can set up a "response to injury," an accelerated form of atherosclerosis that can reblock the artery within a few months. Indeed, angioplasty carries with it a 30 to 50 percent likelihood of repeated blockage—called restenosis—within six months, making necessary either another angioplasty or surgery, or both.

A bulletin from the American Heart Association (May 12, 1993) reported that the professional guidelines for this procedure were not followed *more than 50 percent* of the time. The procedure is very profitable to both cardiologist and the hospital where it is performed; it offers almost immediate (but often short-lived) relief from the pain; and it is fun to do (watching and guiding the catheter on the fluoroscope has been compared to a video game).

What is, I think, most important to bear in mind is that the doctor who performs the angioplasty is usually the one performing the angiogram, thus quite literally making the diagnosis, recommendation, referral, and performing the procedure. (A cartoon in a recent *New Yorker* magazine shows a doctor telling a patient, "That *is* a second opinion. At first, I thought you had something else.") The patient, too, is hardly in a position to exercise judgment as to whether or not to proceed with an angioplasty: he (or she) is stretched out on a table in the operating room with a catheter inserted in his arm (or groin) and must decide soon. It is not exactly a time conducive to reflection.

And—in common with drug and diet therapy—the

risk of heart attack has still not been removed. The risk may be decreased, but by how much is unknown. In my opinion, the purpose of any of these procedures is simply to take care of the problem as best we can and get back to our lives with minimum and easily managed vigilance. Which brings us to:

4. *Surgery—Bypass.* Even after these years there is no more potent phrase to me than "open heart surgery," even though it is misleading: the surgery is performed on the exterior, not the interior, of the heart. This procedure is not without its risks, of course, but all things considered, it is simply one of the truly great miracles of modern science and is in my view the apex of human achievement, the culmination—so far—of the thousands of years of man's efforts to heal his fellow man. If this sounds exaggerated, think of it this way: eleven months after my own surgery (as I write this) I arise at the same time of day I always had before, work as I always had, and have added to my daily routine an hour and a half of fairly rigorous exercise. The health of my heart prevents me from doing nothing I would wish to do and my general health is better than before the surgery—probably, in fact, better than that of most of my peers. Without that surgery I would certainly be an invalid (on guard not to exert myself too much or get excited or stressed) or very possibly dead. Probably the latter.

Hence my enthusiasm.

Miraculous as it is, however, bypass surgery should only be performed in appropriate circumstances. Like angioplasty, the principal criticism leveled against bypass surgery—and justifiably—is that it is performed too frequently. A second opinion from an experienced cardiologist may prevent unnecessary surgery and, in any event, be reassuring. There are no hard and fast rules, but generally angioplasty is the procedure of choice when there is a single blockage high up in an artery, and that artery is not the left anterior descending, or main, artery. Studies have shown bypass surgery to be more effective when the blockage occurs in the left artery and when there is multiple vessel and diffuse disease.

A specific refinement of this recommendation applies to the population of heart disease patients with diabetes under medication (either insulin or oral hypoglycemics), about fifty of whom have bypass surgery or angioplasty in this country *each day*. Among those diabetics with two or more blocked coronary arteries, five-year post-surgical studies have shown bypass surgery to be almost twice as effective as angioplasty, for reasons still not fully explained. But such figures are dramatic indeed and demand attention.

In a British study comparing the success of bypass surgery to a course of medical treatment, a group of 2,649 patients with stable coronary heart disease was split in half: 1,324 had surgery and 1,325 were treated with individually tailored courses of medication, with these results:

1. The surgically treated patients had a reduction in risk of death after five years of *39 percent*.

2. After seven years, the reduction was *32 percent*.

3. After ten years, *17 percent*.

4. Of the drug-treated group, *37 percent* needed surgery anyway.

The patients with the most severe disease derived the greatest benefit from the early surgery.

These are significant numbers and should be borne in mind as you scramble to justify *not* having surgery. The best rule is to grit your teeth and have the surgery if you should, but avoid it like the plague if you shouldn't.

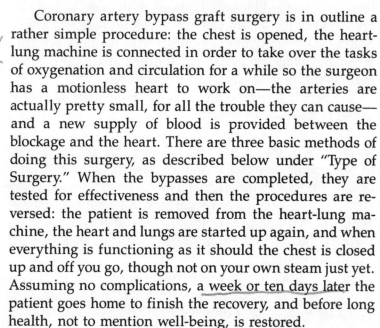

   Coronary artery bypass graft surgery is in outline a rather simple procedure: the chest is opened, the heart-lung machine is connected in order to take over the tasks of oxygenation and circulation for a while so the surgeon has a motionless heart to work on—the arteries are actually pretty small, for all the trouble they can cause—and a new supply of blood is provided between the blockage and the heart. There are three basic methods of doing this surgery, as described below under "Type of Surgery." When the bypasses are completed, they are tested for effectiveness and then the procedures are reversed: the patient is removed from the heart-lung machine, the heart and lungs are started up again, and when everything is functioning as it should the chest is closed up and off you go, though not on your own steam just yet. Assuming no complications, a week or ten days later the patient goes home to finish the recovery, and before long health, not to mention well-being, is restored.

   If that doesn't border on being a miracle I don't know what does.

Causes

The logical question now, of course, is: What causes coronary heart disease? Is it contagious? There are, as it happens, a number of factors involved in causing it. Hardly a day passes without a report in the public press of some new contributor to heart disease, as we can see from the frequency with which we encounter technical words such as "angina," "cholesterol," or "electrocardiogram." One reason for this seeming flood of information is that heart disease is the number one killer in this country, a veritable plague. Another, and more important, reason is that there is something you can do to reduce the likelihood of contracting the disease, diminish its effects, and perhaps even reverse it altogether. By changing your habits you can reduce the chances of its recurrence. You can both prolong and improve the quality of your own life. The better informed you are, and the more preventive steps you take, the more your disease may come under your control. Such a statement can be made about no other health problem of magnitude.

This being the case, it will be wise for us to look at the causes of heart disease, bearing in mind that while we cannot say that any one or combination of these elements *causes* heart disease, we can say that multiple studies have shown that to the greater degree one or more of these factors is present, the greater is the likelihood of disease, and the more factors you have, the greater is the danger from *each* of them. The ten risk factors are:

1. *Heredity.* If both parents have coronary or other vascular disease before age seventy, the increased risk is *200 percent.*

2. *Diabetes.* The presence of diabetes mellitus doubles the risk, or *200 percent.*

3. *Smoking.* Smoking one pack of cigarettes per day or the equivalent increases the risk by *300 percent.*

4. *High Blood Fats.* Often measured only by a relatively high cholesterol level (over 240 milligrams), other factors, such as the ratio of LDL to HDL cholesterol and the level of triglycerides must also be taken into account. This table is worth bearing in mind:

	185	260
Cholesterol level at age 50:	185	260
Heart disease developed within six years:	3/1000	6/1000

5. *Hypertension*. Uncontrolled high blood pressure increases the risk *200 percent*. If the hypertension is under treatment and kept within normal bounds, this factor is basically eliminated.

6. *Sex*. Heart disease is *very rare* among women before menopause. After menopause, women catch up quickly, so that after age sixty-five their risk of having a heart attack or serious disease is about the same as a man's.

7. *Obesity*. Oddly enough, being greatly overweight is not a factor in itself, *but—but, but, but*—it does put a great and unnecessary strain on the heart and reduces the body's ability to fight the disease. Excessive body fat is also associated with high levels of LDL cholesterol, the chief villain in the formation of plaques.

8. *Exercise*. Or more accurately, lack thereof. As in the case of obesity, lack of exercise is not a provable factor. It is certainly true, however, that a reasonable amount of exercise is necessary for good general health. A recommended regimen would be a program that burned two thousand calories a week, about which more later.

9. *Age*. The older you are, male or female, the more likely it is that you will develop heart disease. There is nothing we would care to do about this particular risk factor.

10. *Emotional Stress*. Definitely a factor but unquantifiable. How do you measure the effects of a lawsuit, a tenuous hold on a job, or marital or family problems? What about missing the train, the bus, or the taxi? My suspicion is that this will be shown to be a very important factor, but because of its unmeasurable and indefinable nature, it will remain difficult to prove.

This is probably a good place to report the results of an experiment carried out by cardiologists at Harvard. In a study among people with known coronary heart disease, it was found that arteries not only did not expand with emotional stress (healthy arteries expanded by 10 percent), but actually constricted by 27 percent and this in an *already narrowed* artery. Emotional stress, which increases the heart's need for blood, produces a situation that *decreases* the supply. So in addition to being a possible source of coronary artery disease, it is provably a significant factor in the disease's harmful effects. The image of a man clutching his heart upon receiving tragic news and falling to the ground—felled by a fatal heart attack!—is not an inaccurate one.

Type of Surgery

Starting now, if it has not begun already, the important medical choices will be made by someone else, most notably your cardiologist or other physician. Where and by whom your surgery will take place will be based on your doctor's experience and knowledge, and that's fair enough since that is his or her job. Some knowledge on your part, however, is useful to have, since you always have a veto over these decisions made for you, and some information may be *very* important to have. For instance, it probably doesn't really matter *where* your surgery is done, everything else being equal; but it may matter *what kind* of surgery you have.

There are three methods by which obstructed coronary arteries are bypassed. In the first, one end of a length of vein, usually taken from the saphenous vein in the leg, is sewn, or grafted, into the coronary artery above the blockage—that is to say between the blockage and the heart—and the other end is sewn into the aorta, which as you remember is the large vessel which takes the freshly oxygenated blood from the heart. Occasionally this is also done just as a small loop around the obstruction. Surgically, this type of bypass is fairly simple but *any heart surgery is very complex in itself.* A second method is similar but uses a free length of artery instead. In the third and more recently developed method, one or two lengths of still functioning internal thoracic (formerly known as the internal mammary) artery, or ITA, are dissected away from the wall of the chest, just under the rib cage, and grafted above the blockage. This provides a fresh supply of blood from a new and separate source, whether there is but one surgical graft per bypass or sequential grafts. Surgically, this is a longer and more complex procedure than the vein graft.

Advantages? Disadvantages? Saphenous vein bypasses are quicker and easier to do and the supply of bypass material is more reliable (occasionally the internal thoracic artery is too short to use), and it's preferable to spend less time under anesthesia than more. *But—recent studies have confirmed the experience of doctors that ITA bypasses do not develop new blockages and venous ones frequently do.* The research of Frank H. Sims in New Zealand has shown how the difference in cellular structure between artery and vein produces this immunity from occlusion. Properly performed, which should mean with a surgical microscope with a wide range of magnification (from 4 to 20 power), ITA grafts require reoperation far less often than other methods of this surgery, and then not because of newly developed plaques. By the time you recover from surgery you will have found all of this sufficiently demanding and will have no wish to repeat it—ever. So this is the time for the proverbial ounce of prevention. If your surgeon decides not to perform an ITA bypass procedure there may be a very good reason, but it's worth finding out what that reason is.

Frequently arterial and saphenous vein bypasses are combined, with the arteries used for the more crucial bypasses and the vein for the less important ones. My own surgery was such a combination, and angiography four years later showed the three arterial grafts strong and successful but the venous graft had closed up. Given the choice, I would have preferred *not* to have this example for you, but there you are.

A word about numbers: Your chart will read CABG x 3 or 4 or whatever; this means three or four blockages were or will be bypassed during the surgical procedure, and you will speak of having had three (or however many) bypasses. Let me assure you that four bypasses does not mean the surgical procedure will be twice as rigorous as two!

Choosing a Surgeon

It is unlikely you will have much participation here since your cardiologist probably has developed an excellent working relationship with one or two surgeons, and this rapport in itself has a real value. While it is not important that you have a warm, personal relationship with your surgeon, it *is* important that you trust him or her. For some reason, the notion of "best" has crept into the decisions we make about doctors and will not go away. It is myth. There is no "best" (except for my surgeon, of course). In cardiovascular surgery, as in almost everything else in life, there is the rule of thirds: a third are merely competent (and very rarely less than that), a third are very good, and a third are excellent. The standards in this field are probably as demanding as in any other, so do not be concerned that your surgeon might be a clown.

The mortality rate—the number of patients per hundred whose death is associated with the bypass surgery—

is the relevant statistic for a cardiovascular surgeon. Several states, New York and Pennsylvania among them with more to come, require publication of these numbers. Such publication is controversial, not because there are many incompetent doctors who fear exposure, but because each statistic requires detailed explanation. One doctor may control his statistics by refusing to operate on any but the most favorable cases; another may be willing to risk his statistics for the benefit of truly sick patients in need of his skills; another may be far more skilled and experienced and take on the truly challenging and difficult cases. Since the percentages are extremely small, you can see that the difference of one or two cases can seriously skew the perception of a doctor's ability. So beware of the temptation to rate by these numbers.

A good rule of thumb is the number of procedures a surgeon performs each year. When I think of this, I am always reminded of a friend who spends his summers in a small town in the west (as I do). Suffering much dental pain, he visited the local dentist, who treated him briefly and told him to return the following week; this went on for more than a month, with the procedure being extended each visit. It turned out the dentist was learning the technique *by correspondence course* and was waiting for each new installment. This is unlikely to happen to you.

Between 150 and 200 cases a year is a good number for a surgeon in active practice. Since cardiovascular surgery is a *very* demanding activity, physically, intellectually, and emotionally, it is not unusual for this number to decrease as a surgeon becomes more experienced, and some may work half time or less. But a surgeon who performs only two bypasses annually without work of an equally challenging nature should, I think, be avoided. Similarly, large numbers may indicate a "factory" and not a "tailored" situation. That is not necessarily bad, but is worth looking into.

Choosing a Hospital

While on the subject of *who*, it might be worthwhile to look briefly at *where*. It is not necessary to travel across the country to a famous cardiovascular clinic to have the "best" heart surgeon perform routine bypass surgery. In fact, it's not even a good idea. As a general rule, I would not really recommend flying to some city you do not know, to be surrounded by people with whom you do not have that much in common. While no one is really at home in the hospital, a hospital in your region is more likely to feel comfortable than one far away and, of course, more conducive to visiting by family and maybe a friend. I recall that evocative phrase in the Book of Ruth: "amidst the alien corn." That is how you will feel if you travel far. If you *must*, of course, that is a different story.

A good idea might be to stay within half a day's comfortable travel. There are enough excellent hospitals with very good coronary care centers to make it likely one is close to your home. I suspect that most major, and many not so major, cities in the United States have such hospitals by now. As a rule of thumb, at least a thousand or so bypass surgeries a year should be performed there. Again, this is a decision, or a strong recommendation, that will probably be made by your physician.

One other matter to remember: surgeons work in specific hospitals, so the choices of who and where are made together. Do not expect a surgeon from one hospital to go to another for a routine case.

A note to your friends. Here's a good rule about visiting people you care about who are in the hospital: do it. Don't expect to be entertained by sparkling repartee or a series of hilarious hospital anecdotes, and indeed just plan on seeing your friend asleep. But he (or she) will know you have been there and, at least subconsciously, be very grateful to you for your visit and benefit deeply from the affection you have expressed. Years later, I *still* remember those who came to see me, particularly the unexpected ones.

Besides, isn't it wonderful to be reassured that your friend is still alive? Bet you thought you'd never see the old buzzard again.

□ 4 □

Recovery in the Hospital

There probably is no place in the modern hospital that functions as well as the coronary recovery room or coronary care unit (CCU). Fully staffed twenty-four hours a day and with beds arrayed around the nurse's station, the room defines the word *alert*. Even though patients are attached to a variety of devices that warn of abrupt change in expected patterns, recovery room nurses seem to have a sixth sense of where they are needed *before* they are needed. They also are committed to preserving the dignity and comfort of their patients, two matters which you would think would receive little attention. You may have had an awkward peek in yesterday on your brief orientation tour, but you will find it looks rather different now from your horizontal position.

Here is where you will wake up, more groggy and less in control than you have been almost since infancy, but you are *alive!* You can't exactly jump up in the air and click your heels, but it's over! Back to sleep you go, and you'll wake up sporadically and unpredictably for the next day or two. There will still be a large number of tubes going in and out of you, including a urinary catheter, intravenous tubes connected to needles in your arm for nutrition, two chest drains, a breathing tube, and even one tube in your neck!—but their number will diminish each day. The first to go will be the breathing tube, which will be removed when you can reliably breathe on your own and show this by gagging. This will soon be followed by the two tubes that drain any fluid gathering in your chest, and of whose presence you will be reminded for the rest of your life by two small scars. The scar from the surgery, seemingly six feet long but in fact well short of that, will be bandaged and of no concern to you. What was of real concern to me, however, and something I had not anticipated, was a long incision that had been made in my lower right leg. I subsequently learned that this is the source of the length of vein that is sometimes used as the bypass material and is always ready just in case it is needed. I was prepared for discomfort in my chest but not my leg! A good part of the next week or so was spent crossing my ankles only to have them uncrossed by every passing doctor or nurse.

The doctor will have ordered medication for pain, and your other basic needs will be seen to by the various tubes. For two or three days all those artificial divisions of the day you have so methodically constructed and observed—daytime, nighttime, mealtime, time for bed, time to get up—will cease to have meaning, and you will drift into and out of consciousness without a pattern. Before you know it, you will be up sitting in a chair for brief periods—and don't forget the knocking on the back to loosen up the mucus in your lungs! This always seems to be an intrusion on your peaceful sleep.

The most important thing to bear in mind is to speak up to the nurse or doctor about any discomfort which seems to be unusual. Obviously some discomfort is to be expected and the itching you may feel is from healing tissue; but in spite of all the gauges and meters and other devices you are hooked up to, you are still the best source of information about how you are doing, so make life easier for those taking care of you and tell them about your problems, real or imagined. There is probably an explanation for each of them, and somehow they are less vexing when understood.

Members of your family will be allowed to visit according to the posted schedule. This need not concern you since you are not going anywhere. Besides, it is important to remember that these visits are for *them*, not you; while you have been sleeping peacefully and getting more healthy, *they* have been worried sick. They are the ones who need to see that you are alive and mending well; you already know it. By the way, the shock you may see in their faces is probably caused by you: unless some miracle has occurred, you look terrible.

I was trying to think of a way to describe how you will feel and the only thing I came up with is that it is like having been hit full force by a truck (not that I speak from experience), without the experience of the accident itself. You will be stunned from the trauma of the surgery and your chest will feel as though it's been crushed. You have suffered from exposure in a way (your body temperature was lowered during the surgery) and you went through severe emotional trauma—and yet what you will find surprising is the absence of pain. Just take it easy, sleep as much as you can, don't worry about anything, and ask for more medication if you get too uncomfortable. The only work you have to do is with that seemingly silly little toylike apparatus for your breathing. Pneumonia is now your biggest enemy, and your best defense is getting your lungs strong again.

On the third day after surgery, when you are awake as much as asleep, able to get from your bed to your chair reasonably well, and the tubes branching from you are diminishing in number, you will return to your room to begin the next stage of your recovery. It is quite a shock, leaving a place bustling with activity most of the day for the relative tranquility of your room. Now is the time to start pushing yourself: rather than stay in bed and watch television all day, get up and walk as much as you can— around your room at first, then out in the corridor, then take longer and longer expeditions. It is unlikely that you will still have any tubes, but if you do, they can probably be fixed to go along with you. It's important to remember that you are *not* sick, that you are not afflicted with illness as are most patients in the hospital. You are someone recovering your strength after major surgery, and you need to return to an active life as soon as you can. So get out there! For me, the best part of this time was being able to go to the bathroom by myself. Also, I felt a lot better when I put on street clothes for my walks down hospital corridors; they asserted my status as healthy and recovering, as opposed to being ill, a patient. Even with this activity, though, my appetite was small and unenthusiastic, which was unlike me. This too would change—with a vengeance.

By now you will have become familiar with your new scar, which is probably painted with antiseptic daily and kept loosely bandaged. Your rib cage was spread wide and later sewn together with stainless-steel wire, so it would be strange if you did not feel some discomfort. My sternum, the front of the chest, felt it would split if I twisted in the wrong way, but of course it did not. It did, however, click occasionally when I moved, and that was a little disconcerting. At any rate, like any broken bone, it heals fairly quickly, in, say, four to six weeks, and in that time your scar will be healed, too. A useful trick is to clutch a pillow to your chest while talking to friends, especially if there is danger of being amused. Laughing can be quite uncomfortable, but don't avoid it just for comfort's sake. Like the old joke about the arrow-pierced soldier who survived at the Little Big Horn, it only hurt when I laughed.

During your remaining time in the hospital—this will vary from three to seven days, depending on your rate of recovery and the policy of your hospital and/or surgical insurance plan—the dietician will visit you to discuss your new diet. We will talk more about this later on, but you'd better get used to the idea that life is going to change dramatically in the food department. Since you have been given a new lease on life by your surgeon, the least you can do is take proper care of the new equipment. Besides, even though this hospital experience was not as bad as you had anticipated, you can take my word that it's really not something you want to do again.

By now your chest numbness will have faded to a constant tingling sensation—what someone I interviewed called a ginger ale chest. This will continue for a long time, before fading away after some weeks. Of course it's only all that tissue healing and nerves sorting themselves out, so it's a sign of health. But report any sensations that don't feel normal: an infection can start very small and change, or end, your life in no time.

The five to seven days before you go home should be spent walking as much as you can and resting, and there will be a few more tests of various types, including an echocardiogram (a picture of your heart made by sound waves), to measure the success of the surgery and monitor your progress. This is the period during which pericarditis might appear. You may remember the pericardium as the envelope of tissue that surrounds and protects the heart. It seems to resent being handled, as it had to be during surgery, and it may have an artery or two through it. Sometimes—in about one patient in ten—it becomes inflamed and less supple than normal. (Indeed, it is often so much less supple that you can *feel* it rubbing against the heart, and it can be heard through the stethoscope.) I was one of the rare few to contract this condition and would have passed it up gladly. Anti-inflammatory drugs are used to treat it and in me the side effects were most unpleasant: I would wake up in the middle of the night soaked with perspiration and of course shivering from the resultant chill. I felt almost degraded somehow, as though I had wet my bed. How thankful I was for the cheerful night nurse who looked after me and made my bed afresh! A friend to whom I described waking up in a pool of salt water inquired if I were also singing sea chanteys.

Occasional blood tests during this period monitor such an inflammation and any possible infection as well; they also reveal the hematocrit level, the ratio of blood cells to liquid plasma. Normal levels are around 45 percent, but it is not unusual for this to be cut in half by all that has been going on. Although efforts were made to preserve as much blood as possible during your surgery, many cells were lost or damaged and intravenous supplements have taken up the space those cells used to occupy. In addition, the many blood samples you have provided for testing have taken their toll. Blood cells take time to regenerate and until they do you may feel even more weak and tired. This will make exercise less attractive, of course, but it is still important. Transfusions could speed up the process, but prudence would dictate caution in their use. Virulent (and often deadly) hepatitis and the AIDS virus are passed by transfusion, and while modern screening processes can usually detect such perils, we know absolutely that no transfusion will transmit no infection.

After seven or eight days of less frequent tests, more frequent exercise, and independence from tubes, and about the time you start to get restless, it will be time to go home. I lived only a few miles from the hospital and my trip home was made easy by my friends John and Claudia, who listened to none of my protests and took a bright and cold Saturday morning off to drive in from the country and bundle me and my meager possessions into their car. If you live far from the hospital, plan to make your journey in stages of no more than three or four hours each if by car—get out and take a walking break periodically—and if you are flying, walk in the airport but try to have use of a wheelchair if you should need it. You may have felt like some sort of Goliath by the time you were ready to leave the hospital, but believe me you are not, as you will soon discover. The idea is to get home reasonably quickly, but don't kill yourself in the process. A good rule to follow is that you will be able to do about half what you think you can. Don't push it!

Important Self Care!

❑ 5 ❑

Recovery at Home

It would be nice to think of the recuperation period at home as a continuation of the last week in the hospital, but that is not the case. Since the diagnosis of your disease, or at least since you were told of the need for surgery, you have been caught up in the whole virtual frenzy of denial, acceptance, fear, anxiety, and preparation; then as a patient your mind and will virtually went on hold. In the hospital you did as you were told, accepting the status of passive participant known as "patient." Now you are home, in familiar territory, and all the other is behind you. It is the moment you have been praying for—that whole damn *very* unpleasant thing is over! The relief, at first, is great. Sometimes being home like this can make you almost believe the rest did not happen. It did. This is the first day of the rest of your life, and things are going to be very different, on almost every front.

There are few hard and fast rules for this period but here are some important ones:

Do not drive a car or similar vehicle for a month. As much as you might feel otherwise, your coordination and reaction time are not what they were and need time to return. If you should have an accident, the chest cannot provide as much protection to the heart as it can with a healed sternum. Ancillary to this is the suggestion that you stop, get out and stretch, and preferably *take a brief walk every hour or two if you take a long car trip* as a passenger. Your body really needs it.

Do not lift anything weighing ten pounds or more for ten weeks. This one is obvious. Your sternum needs as much stability and rest as it can get while it heals and lifting is not conducive to proper healing. Don't even *think* about lifting those groceries or golf clubs or granddaughter or girlfriend or whatever.

Be vigilant about swelling in your legs, particularly the leg that offered up the section of saphenous vein. You were probably given a pair of support stockings in the hospital, and you should continue to wear them, or Ace bandages, should you need them. Walk as much as you can. When you sit, raise your legs and rest them at hip level. Fluid can collect easily, accumulate painlessly, and very quickly cause serious trouble. A little bit of care and attention goes a very long way.

Resume your daily routine of getting up, shaving, showering or bathing, dressing (in comfortable clothes) *every day.* You'll feel much better than if you lounge around in bed. Your chest scar can get wet now that a scab has formed, but keep the scab dry and only loosely bandaged so that it can dry out. Keep your leg scar ultra clean and it should heal quickly with no problem.

Start your new diet unless there is a reason not to, such as anemia. With so many other changes in your life this will seem to be a small one, and before you know it you will not only be used to it, you will prefer it.

Call your doctor immediately if you feel something is really not as it should be: increased body temperature, unusual pulse, nausea, any new and unfamiliar pain,

shortness of breath—indeed, anything unusual or unexpected. And if you are not *absolutely sure* about timing or
dosage of your medication, find out immediately. It is
likely you will be aware of your medicine *only* if you take it
improperly or not at all.

And a tip to end on: sleeping propped up on your back
in a semi-reclining position takes a night or two to get
accustomed to, but in the long run helps you to avoid
hours of discomfort and sleeplessness.

It is important to remember that the recovery of
strength does not pick up where you left off in the
hospital. I had been able to walk to the far reaches of a
large hospital and return to my room ready for more
activity, but the "hothouse" environment of the hospital is
very different from the real world. Get outside and walk,
yes, but calculate your limits and stick to them. I went out
for a walk my second or third afternoon home, got four
blocks from my house, and lost it; I had to take a taxi
home. I did not even feel ashamed. This reduced strength
may be a result of all the unrecognized extra activities and
strains of an average day—such as getting dressed, climb-
ing stairs, planning ahead—which are not present in a
hospital day, but I think there is something larger. You
have spent much of your life building up your stamina,
your vigor, your capacity to endure, and now it is gone,
whether stolen by the surgery, the prolonged anesthesia,
or the emotional strain of it all. Whatever the reason, it is
gone. You have always had something to fall back on
when you needed it, and now you don't have any reserves
of energy. Someone has robbed that bank where you kept
your savings. You can bemoan its loss, which does you no
good at all, or you can get on with life. You will probably
find, if you have not already, that the time comes when

you simply cannot push yourself further. Don't try, whether to accommodate the needs of others or to salve your own pride. It won't work.

There is a cure! The first thing you must do is assess your own limits and stay within them. Be selfish—but don't get too used to it! Let visitors leave while you still enjoy them, not when they have worn you out. Don't try to control everything around you; the world got along without you when you were in the hospital and probably can for a bit longer. Don't be reluctant to ask for help (but don't overdo it, either). Don't take on new responsibilities or projects just yet—there is more on your plate than you are aware of. Take naps when you feel the urge: just lie down on the couch or the floor and sleep. This is a very useful skill to acquire if you don't already have it, and one you will use for years to come. Above all, and in all things, pace yourself.

In many ways, what I'm about to tell you is the crux of this book. Those who have not experienced what *we* have undergone can tell you about symptoms and blood tests and surgical procedures, diets and exercise and recovery programs. What we know about is the effects of these things, and they can be unexpectedly powerful as you will learn when you go through them. First, of course, is the gratitude you feel for your doctor and family and those who took care of you, yes, but as much or more for just being alive. Every minute, every experience, takes on a hitherto unknown intensity and the simplest things produce a joy that is almost painful. This period in my life was what the English call the Run Up to Christmas, and the sight of children dressed up for Christmas events, the sound of holiday music, the festive air of New York, and the power of the Christmas message stretched my emotional capacity to its limits. Never had I felt such love for those near me—my son, my maybe new girlfriend, and a few close personal friends. Never have I since. Many a cough hid a catch in my throat, many a tear was secretly brushed away. New York was cold and windy that year, so I was able to hide my humanity well.

For some reason anger appears, too. Exactly why this happens I don't know, but it does. The anger may come from a variety of sources. You have been through a lot, it is true, and you may think your ordeal was unfair (actually you've been lucky, but never mind). Another cause may be the dimensions, the enormity of the shock you've experienced, and your emotions are only now catching up. The physical shock of prolonged surgery, of the anesthesia, of the healing process you are going through, may play its part. I can't help but think that the strong proof of your own mortality and vulnerability, together with the loss of control over your own destiny, is also powerful, especially considering how invulnerable you felt just a short time ago. After all, you are still young! But you have seen the handwriting on the wall, and it scared you.

The manifestations of this anger may appear out of proportion to whatever triggers it; its appearance may well alarm those who know you well and care about you, your family especially, and they may think that the person they sent off to the hospital with such love and apprehension has somehow stayed there, to be replaced by an angry and unpredictable grouch. It's important that they know this anger is part of the whole package and will go away eventually; make sure they see it as part of your recovery and not a permanent condition.

I hope you're ready for this one! Often—not always, but frequently—considerable memory loss occurs. A face may seem familiar but you are unable to put a name to it; what should be a well-known story among family or friends may seem unfamiliar; things you obviously knew may seem to disappear. I was setting the dinner table on Christmas with an old friend and was unable to remember the name of one of the standard utensils—in fact I had *no* idea what it was called—and had to do some subtle manipulating of the conversation to get her to produce the name (it was a spoon). My son maintained that I had always been forgetful and that I was not then any worse than I had been, but never mind. Be prepared for and accept these lapses; don't let them upset you, and, indeed, get what you can out of them. I was able to listen to a stream of old jokes and stories from a particularly outrageous friend, who protested he had told me all of them before. I had no memory of them and enjoyed every word. This lapse in your memory will either improve or you will learn to live with it.

Strangely enough, the anger and forgetfulness have an unlikely companion: compassion. Those people—usually the old or infirm—whose deliberate pace often makes us impatient, sometimes to the point of rudeness, are now seen with more understanding and empathy. We too must now take our time—what's the rush? Unfortunately this attitude of compassion and pity is the first to disappear on the road back to normality.

To return to the subject of anger during your recuperation, if your family is informed about that anger and its source, you should leave little damage in your wake. Normally it doesn't last too long—except possibly for the effects on those who bear its force.

A famous American corporation executive, a man of great power, recently underwent a bypass operation that was widely reported in the press. When it was announced that he was returning to work almost immediately after the surgery—I think it was about six days—I had two reactions. The first was a statement to my wife that *something* was going to happen, and soon. Sure enough, within days, his second in command, almost his alter ego, was summarily fired. My second reaction was, where the hell was his doctor? Why didn't he lock his patient up for a while? Sometimes it's best to just get potential trouble off the streets, if only briefly. The answer, of course—I mean about his doctor's whereabouts—is that his surgeon was monitoring the results of his surgery, and his cardiologist had a sharp eye on the condition of his heart and his health in general. Emotional health got the short end of the stick, as it usually does. It is important for you to be vigilant about this.

One of the most important developments in medicine in this century has been the gradual realization that emotional and mental health are identical to physical health in the sense that identifiable illnesses have sources, symptoms, specific treatments and, frequently, cures. They are not indications of evil or moral decay; recognizing them and acknowledging them is not escapist or cowardly. It is essential.

I bring this up here because there is an illness that is often associated with heart surgery and is frequently overlooked: depression. I have seen published estimates of the frequency of this disorder that run as high as 30 percent. But my own experience—in talking to patients in hospitals or elsewhere, as well as "veterans" in social situations or Mended Hearts meetings—would suggest a rate of twice that, or more.

It is not surprising that this illness is so closely linked to heart disease, particularly since it was long believed that the heart was the source and seat of moods. Like heart disease itself, the symptoms of depression are similar to those of other problems and are easily disguised; we are all reluctant to admit to them and skillful at avoiding the identification. And like heart disease, depression is a specific illness, subject to treatment and possible cure. Unlike heart disease, however, we have no equivalent of angiography to identify the nature and extent of the involvement.

It is inevitable that you will feel some of the signs and symptoms of depression as a result of your surgery: sadness, as if from a loss; gloomy, negative thinking; diminished expectations of self or others; diminished self-esteem; profound feelings of self-doubt; inappropriate feelings of guilt; unreasonable fear of death; loss of pleasure and interest in things you enjoyed before; and thoughts of suicide. Physical symptoms may be fatigue and loss of energy; reluctance and refusal to participate in physical activities; weight loss from a diminished appetite; decreased sexual desire (often from fear); and a change in sleeping habits. Distinguishing the disease of depression from legitimate and appropriate feelings of sadness following surgery will be determined by intensity and duration. Actual events can also cause some of these conditions, further complicating identification. For instance, I was defrauded of a large sum of money by someone I not only trusted but considered a friend, and you can imagine the effects *that* had on my recovery. Prescribed drugs may also cloud the issue because some whose role is to moderate and regulate the heartbeat also act as a general depressant. The class of drugs known as beta-blockers is sometimes a culprit here. And just to complicate matters more, the need for bypass surgery often coincides with (or causes or is caused by?) a man's mid-life crisis—what is sometimes called male menopause.

We men in our forties, fifties, and sixties, the population most likely to need bypass surgery, were raised to suppress our emotional awareness and needs and be "men." This may have served your needs as a young man, and perhaps you were able to get away with it for a while, but now some change is likely to be required. Heart disease will kill you unless you bring it under control; depression is just as insidious when left uncontrolled. It can rob you of your life, from within, quietly sapping your strength, your will, your joy, your identity. Unfortunately, there are many who never recover from their surgery and become "cardiac cripples."

Vigilance is essential, for depression is very wily; not only can it appear in many guises, it can also *rob you of your will to do anything about it*. The question "What's the point? What can be done, anyway?" is almost a surefire means of identifying the disease.

Exactly what causes the root problem I can't say with certainty, but we're not lacking for candidates: fear of another heart attack; hints of mortality; reduction (usually temporary) of strength and stamina; loss of control over our lives. It may well be that the effects of prolonged anesthesia are more profound than we know, and the suggestion that the lowering of the blood's temperature (by about 10 degrees Centigrade or 18 degrees Fahrenheit) during surgery is responsible for depression may well have merit. Whatever the cause or causes, some people just never make it back to a real life, deciding to hunker down in this netherworld of gloom, self-doubt, and reluctance to act. I know; I fight it every day, sometimes successfully but sometimes not.

Depression *may* be as easy to treat as it is difficult to identify. Moods are caused by chemicals in your brain called neurotransmitters. If you have an improper balance or deficit of one of these chemicals, there will be an effect, just as there would be with an imbalance in the chemistry of your digestive system, say, or your blood. *Chemical imbalances in your brain are no different.*

If I have a single plea for you it is this: don't try to tough it out. It won't work. If you are making the required changes in your life as times goes by and are *still* not feeling better but maybe even feel worse, it's time to talk to your physician about it and seek treatment. Something as simple as daily medication may be as important to the restoration of the quality of your life as was the elaborate surgical procedure you underwent.

After heart surgery, some people make the decision to alter their lives completely. This decision may be motivated by depression, but more often is not. Many who have spent their years in pursuit of the almighty dollar decide to enjoy life while they can; many see the material grind as joyless; many decide to spend more time with the family they ignored for so long; many pursue a stronger commitment to life or to their faith or to a new career, seeing this dividend of time as a second chance at life and their last chance at fulfillment. Choices in this category are just that, choices, decisions made, not avoided, and so are an expression of a decision to act as opposed to deciding *not* to act. Behavior stemming from the need to make changes can be as traumatic as the effects of depression, but it can also be *very* exciting. I started a whole new life after surgery, and it included a marriage; a stronger awareness of my faith and the love I feel for my wife and son, and also a new son; more time spent doing the things I love, particularly fishing; a greater enjoyment in the company of my friends; an intensified response to art; and sometimes even a greater tolerance for people.

Now if only the depression could be dealt with successfully.

I have saved the best news in this chapter for last.
Immediately after heart surgery sex is fantastic. At first I
thought it was just me, but when I spoke with others I
found it to be almost universally true. I don't know if this
is because sex is the activity that essentially defines life, or
because your emotions are so close to the surface at that
vulnerable time, or because you need to feel close to
someone because you have felt so alone, or if there is some
physical reason. But wow! As with any other form of
exercise, your stamina is limited, but the widespread
concern of heart surgery causing impotence is without
foundation; many medications will do that, but that is
another story. For now, don't worry about it.

Heart surgery is different, I think, from any other
surgery, in that it seems to involve the very core of your
being, virtually your soul. You can watch people comparing their experiences of knee surgery, say, or hip replacement, or gallbladder removal, and they speak with a
distance and disinterest you would think more appropriate for business matters or cars. It is as though other
medical events take place without touching you deeply,
but heart surgery is of cosmic significance. You will
probably feel this intensity for some time and wish to
describe your case to anyone who will listen, maybe even
write a book about it. Don't worry, though; by the time
you have told everyone you know, and some you don't,
your compulsion will have begun to fade.

In the meantime, you will have become aware of the
importance of the heart in contemporary thought and the
frequency of reference to it.

The Heart in Contemporary Mythology

Hearty
Heartfelt
Heartless
Heartrending
Heartache
Heartbroken
Heartsick
Heartland
Heart-stopping
Heartburn
Heart and soul
At heart.

Put one's heart into it
After my own heart
With all my heart
To have the heart
Have a heart!
From the heart.

Take to heart
Wear one's heart on one's
  sleeve
(Zing went the) strings of my
  heart
Heart to heart
Heart of my heart
Heart of stone.

Hearts and flowers
Hearts (the card game)
Hearts (the card suit)
Learn by heart
Heart of the matter
Give or lose one's heart to
Near one's heart
Lose heart

Sweetheart.

❑ 6 ❑

Life, Part II

After you have been home a few weeks and are beginning to wonder if all these events *really* took place—and I hope you have indulged yourself a bit (but not too much) during this time—it will be time to assess the situation and think about something you probably thought you had lost: your future. We will forgive your carelessness about your life-style the first time around because you didn't *really* know the consequences, but now you not only know them, you have suffered them. It would be nice to think that this heart disease is like appendicitis—you had a problem, it was dealt with, and now no more aggravation—but such is not the case. What you have had is a warning, and what you have been given is a second chance. What you do with it is up to you.

Short of being hit by lightning or a runaway oxcart, you have a long future before you, one in which you have an advantage over most of your fellow mortals: after all, you have met the enemy and came out ahead *this* time. If you're lucky, you have learned that dying is not all it's cracked up to be. It is essential to remember that you still have heart disease, though, and are *more* likely to suffer its consequences now than before because you're older and more vulnerable to it. So it is time to begin Life II.

Welcome! You gave us quite a scare there for a while! We're glad to have you with us. May your stay be a long and happy one. Do you recall the list of risk factors we looked at—probably skimmed—a while back? It is time to review them in detail. We looked at them then as probable sources of our heart disease, and now we will look at them as guides to how we must change our lives in order to avoid further difficulties.

Let's take them in order.

1. *Heredity.* Unless you are reading this in its four thousandth edition, there is still no method by which we can change our parents or grandparents, nor do we have any need to try to predict the likelihood of our contracting heart disease, so let's pass this one by.

2. *Diabetes.* Again, there's not a lot you can do; you either have diabetes mellitus or you don't. If you do, take particular care and follow your doctor's orders.

3. *Smoking.* We saw earlier that smoking one pack of cigarettes per day increases the risk of heart disease 300 percent. Now we have a simple rule: don't. Period. End of story.

Smoking is what I was most worried about. I had not given up cigarettes before, as so many do, frequently, but of course had heard dreadful stories of the grip that nicotine had on smokers. I was curious to see that I was experiencing no yearning for tobacco, even back home with all the prompting hints: telephone, typewriter, a drink before dinner, conversation after. Perhaps I had undergone the physical withdrawal during the several days I was zonked out; perhaps I was subconsciously aware of the unspoken pact I had with my heart surgeon (and dear friend); perhaps I had finally accepted how harmful cigarette smoking is. But even though I still felt weak and frail, I think I was reveling in my new health. I know I was constantly aware of being able to breathe in more deeply than ever before, to discover a distant part of my lungs (or so it seemed) I had not known was there. It was like being a teenager again, running in the spring air! Add to this the knowledge that every day after the surgery was a dividend to my life, and you have not only a convert but also one who is keen on getting out the message:

Don't smoke cigarettes! I do smoke a good cigar, a very good cigar, three or four times a year now, to be honest, but I do not inhale it. And for heaven's sake, don't tell my doctor!

4. *High blood fats.* This subject requires a lot of our attention and so I have decided to devote a chapter to it.

5. *Hypertension.* This also gets a chapter to itself, but in the meantime, let's remember that hypertension, or uncontrolled high blood pressure, increases risk 200 percent. Even had this condition gone undetected before your surgery, it is known and being treated now. As with diabetes, take your medication *and* the other orders from your doctor that go with it.

6. *Sex.* Another factor beyond our control. Even if you had a sex change operation you would have none of those female sex hormones that work so well against heart disease. Sorry.

7. *Obesity.* This is like the risk of smoking cigarettes: you have complete control. There are no secrets and no panaceas. Lose weight. Now.

8. *Exercise.* If you have not exercised *regularly* before your surgery, now is the time to start. Some suggestions follow.

9. *Age.* This is the risk factor we are doing everything in our power to *increase*.

10. *Emotional stress.* The great mystery, the great un-quantifiable; like Justice Potter Stewart—one of those very rare Republican appointments to the Supreme Court of real stature—said about pornography, "I don't know what it is, but I know it when I see it." What is stressful to some people is essential to others, of course, but there are some reliable generalities to reduce stress: learn to relax, by prayer or meditation or deep breathing or biofeedback or music or reading or visualization. Focus your attentions on achievable goals, not unrealistic ones. It is too late for you to pitch Game One of the World Series. As much as dealing with stress is important, it is also wise to *avoid* it: stay away from those situations and people that you *know* are going to drive you up the wall. The two rules, then, are:

a. Identify the sources of stress in *your* life.
b. *Avoid* those where possible.

Now let's return to the first subject that we postponed, high blood fats. For us that basically takes the form of cholesterol, a word we see every day and about whose nature we must learn more.

□ 7 □

Cholesterol

There are two substances which are essential to the body's chemistry but which are also the stuff of arterial plaques: *triglycerides* and *cholesterol*. The second you have heard and read a lot about and will soon read more; the first may not be quite as familiar. Current studies are revealing its role in plaque formation.

Glucose is the "fuel" for the body's growth and energy, and excess glucose—along with other products of digestion—is converted to fatty acids which in turn are stored as triglycerides. They are formed directly from the products of digestion, what you eat. We think of them as "fat," both what we see on red meat and what seems to grow too quickly around our middle. Recent studies have shown that elevated levels can increase the risk of heart attack, seemingly because these molecules contribute to the formation of small and medium-sized plaques. It is the progressive growth of such plaques that leads to a heart attack. Further, it has been learned that this activity takes place even in conditions of high levels of HDL (good) cholesterol and low levels of LDL (bad) cholesterol. So it is becoming clear that triglycerides can be bad guys, too. But take heart! Their levels can be *completely* controlled by diet and exercise.

Cholesterol would be the one-word reply of most people

if they were asked to name the chief cause of heart disease. That, of course, makes it a villain, a poisonous substance. Yet it is an essential part of the body's chemistry. Does this make sense? Yes and no. And much else about it amounts to shades of yes and no, good and bad. Let's see if we can sort it out.

Chemically, cholesterol is classified as a steroid; it is yellowish and has an oily/fatty consistency, not unlike a thinner candle wax, and is found in all animal fats—milk and milk products (cheese), meat, and eggs. It is also manufactured in the body, particularly in the liver, to the degree that you would have enough for your own needs even if you never again consumed food containing cholesterol. A 180-pound man contains about half a pound of it, concentrated in the brain and spinal cord. Cholesterol is one of the essential building elements of the human body and is necessary for the manufacture of:

1. cell membranes
2. myelin (the sheathing of axons, nerve fibers)
3. bile (necessary for the digestion of fats)
4. vitamin D (necessary for calcium metabolism)
5. sex hormones.

Levels of cholesterol in the blood are determined by heredity and by diet, and are regulated by the liver. As fats, particularly saturated fats, are digested and enter the bloodstream, the liver removes them for excretion. If the levels of saturated fat are too high, the liver is unable to remove all of them; when levels are low, a healthy liver deals with them successfully. The liver converts cholesterol into bile acids which it then secretes into the intestine. If the diet is sufficiently high in soluble fiber (oats, bran or meal, beans, several fruits), the fiber absorbs the bile acids and excretes them; if not, the acids are reabsorbed and added to the body's cholesterol pool, thereby becoming available for other purposes.

Like oil in water, cholesterol does not dissolve in blood and so is carried to the tissues on complex structures called chylomicrons. These also carry triglycerides, lipoproteins, and an apoprotein (which eases the chemical process of mixing with the blood). As your doctors have doubtless pointed out, cholesterol will also drop off this structure and accumulate on the wall of the artery, contributing to the formation of the atheroma or plaque which, as we learned earlier, is the cause of the blockage.

Now there are two types of this cholesterol-carrying molecule, low density lipoprotein or LDL and high density lipoprotein or HDL. (There is in fact a third, very low density, or VLDL, but that is of the same character as the LDL and need not concern us further.) The LDL molecule tends to deposit cholesterol on artery walls at suitable sites and is therefore the vehicle for the problem; the HDL molecule, on the other hand, will pick up excess cholesterol and move it along through the system for eventual excretion.

A number of studies have shown comparatively high levels of LDL cholesterol among people who exercise little if at all and have diets high in fat and smoke cigarettes, while those who exercise regularly, consume much less fat, and do not smoke have higher levels of HDL cholesterol. *The incidence of heart disease is much higher among the former group.*

One of those blood tests to which you are regularly subjected measures the amount of cholesterol in your blood; the measurements are of milligrams of cholesterol per 100 milliliters (or deciliter) of plasma (liquid), and the result is expressed in a single number, which is the sum of two numbers, the levels of HDL and LDL. The LDL level is invariably higher than the HDL, and normal amounts are in the range of 150 to 180 total cholesterol with a desired HDL level of at least 45; this would leave normal levels of LDL between 105 and 135. While the total level is significant, so is the ratio—the proportion—of total cholesterol to HDL.

For example, say your total cholesterol is 200, with an LDL level of 150 and an HDL of 50. The ratio of total cholesterol to HDL would therefore be 200:50 or 4:1, and this in turn is expressed as a decimal, 4.0. *The greater the proportion of HDL cholesterol to total cholesterol, the lower the ratio decimal.* Recently published studies confirm earlier indications of a direct relationship between lower cholesterol ratio decimals and decreased frequency of heart disease. *The higher the amount of HDL cholesterol, the less likelihood there is of heart disease.* Here are the numbers.

3.5 or lower	least risk
3.5–4.4	below average
4.5–6.4	average
6.5–13.4	high risk
13.5 or greater	highest risk

Which leads us to the following simplification.

GOOD: total cholesterol to HDL cholesterol ratio of *4.5 or less.*
BAD: total cholesterol to HDL cholesterol ratio of *6.5 or more.*

I'm not providing all this just for your edification, mind you; while it is important to know why you are where you are, it is even more important to know that since you have heart disease you must make every effort to keep its effects to a minimum. Now you will have to go on a cholesterol watch, which means keeping the total cholesterol below 200 and the HDL ratio below 4.5.

Let's see how this can be done.

A recent theory suggests how LDL cholesterol becomes "outlaw." The body produces unstable products called reactive oxygen species, some of which are oxygen free-radicals. These can be thought of as people desperate for a date for Saturday night, what chemists call unstable, and they hunt desperately for a molecule to attach themselves to, a process called oxidation. If that oxidation takes place in the LDL molecule, it changes in nature, much like butter becomes rancid in air, and attaches itself to the cells of the arterial wall as the first step in the development of a plaque.

With the discovery of this process goes a possible solution: substances called antioxidants inhibit the oxidation, and some studies have shown that large doses (160 times normal!) of vitamin E do just that. Carotene and riboflavin are also effective, and vitamin C either works, too, or enhances the effects of the others.

But not even the most enthusiastic proponents of Vitamin E suggest that it alone is sufficient to control cholesterol levels in your body. For that, more active steps are required, and we'll examine those after a brief look at a real bad guy lurking in the wings.

□ **8** □

The Silent Killer

There is another disease so closely associated with heart disease that the two are often seen as one: their symptoms often overlap, they provoke and contribute to each other, they may arise from similar sources. They are fellow killers, far worse than any who ever stalked the streets of the Old West, and between them they account for many more than a million deaths each year. That disease is hypertension, high blood pressure, and is not the same as nervous tension, with which it is often confused. It is particularly dangerous because its symptoms and effects are quiet—and often lethal.

Blood pressure is just that: the force of the stream of blood against the walls of the main arteries. If the force is too great it can roughen those walls, thus providing a "seat" or suitable foundation for the accumulation of atheroma material. The arterial walls may also weaken, becoming prone to rupture, which is why stroke, blindness, kidney damage, and heart attacks are associated with hypertension. Blood pressure is measured in millimeters of mercury (mm/Hg) with the aid of a sphygmomanometer, which is that familiar cuff, air pump, and thermometer–looking instrument, and is represented by two numbers, expressed as some number over some number. The first number, the higher of the two, measures the systolic pressure or pressure during systole, when the ventricles are contracting and expelling blood from the heart; the second records the pressure when the ventricles relax and refill, a period called diastole, and is called the diastolic pressure.

Generally accepted ranges are:

Normal	Lower Range of Hypertension	Danger
120/80	140/90	160/95

Large population studies have also shown the following:

Diastolic pressure	<80	80–89	>90
Risk	minimum	moderate	higher
Population affected (U.S.)	41%	34%	25%

One American in four suffers from high blood pressure!

Blood pressure is raised by one or more of three causes: the retaining of water by the kidneys, thereby increasing the amount of fluid in the body; constriction, by heart disease or other cause, of the arteries; and the heart pumping with greater than usual force (as it does during exercise). Even if mild, hypertension should be treated—it usually responds very well to treatment—and the method of treatment is not important so long as it is effective. Here are the principal methods:

1. If overweight, lose weight.

2. Stop smoking.

3. Decrease alcohol consumption.

4. Reduce salt intake (salt causes the body to retain fluid).

5. Exercise.

6. Relax.

7. Adhere to an appropriate drug therapy.

Types of drugs are:

1. diuretics
2. ACE (angiotensin-converting enzyme) inhibitors
3. alpha-blockers
4. beta-blockers
5. calcium channel-blockers

Diuretics. These drugs increase the volume of urine produced by the kidneys, thus promoting excretion of salts and water.

ACE inhibitors. Short for angiotensin—converting enzyme inhibitors. This class of drugs acts to prevent the production of angiotensin II, a hormone that constricts blood vessels, thereby slowing blood flow.

Alpha-blockers. Short for alpha-adrenergic blocking drugs. When stimulated, the alpha receptors in arteries and veins cause the vessels to dilate, or constrict. This class of drugs prevents that, thereby promoting vascular relaxation and easier blood flow.

Beta-blockers. Beta-adrenergic blocking drugs. During exercise or emotional stress, hormones are released that stimulate the heart's beta receptors to pump harder. By blocking the responses to these receptors, these drugs reduce the output of blood from the heart and thereby decrease blood pressure.

Calcium channel-blockers. These are a new class of drugs with a very sophisticated mechanism. In order to constrict, muscles must have calcium. These drugs block the passage of calcium into the muscle cells that control the diameter of blood vessels, thus preventing arterial muscles from constricting. Procardia XL is a particularly effective drug for relieving angina and reducing blood pressure. It is, however, very expensive.

Some of these drugs are also of use in treating heart disease and its symptoms, such as angina pectoris. You will find an extensive list of drugs in the chapter devoted to medications. It is of particular importance because people respond to these drugs differently, and you may need to change and mix and match before you find the combination that works best for you. It is essential that you be an active participant in determining the best course of treatment for yourself.

Because hypertension is so widespread—about one in four Americans has it—it has been widely studied, and because it responds so well to treatment, the results of those studies are very dramatic. Here are two of them: in a study of about 11,000 subjects with diastolic pressure above 90, 50 percent were treated with drugs and 50 percent had other, traditional therapy. After five years there was a 20 percent reduction overall *and* 45 percent fewer deaths from stroke, 46 percent fewer deaths from heart attack than would have been expected—*but*, among the drug-treated half there were 17 percent fewer deaths overall, 45 percent fewer stroke deaths, and 26 percent fewer heart attack deaths.

In the TOMHS, the Treatment of Mild Hypertension Study, 902 people with mild hypertension, that is, with a diastolic pressure between 90 and 99, were studied over five years. When any one of the five standard drug types was added to a basic diet and exercise routine, heart attack risk fell by 31 percent against a group with the same regimen and no drugs.

Hypertension, like heart disease, can be brought under control but not cured. Since you have heart disease, it is altogether likely you have hypertension, too, and you can learn to live with it. Within a few months of your surgery, begin to work with your doctor to develop a comfortable regimen to bring hypertension under control. Be particularly vigilant toward the side effects of drugs, for some can be quite unpleasant and insidious (impotence is not at all infrequent), and report *all* of them. There is a very wide spectrum of types of drugs and choices within those types, and the drug or combination that works with a minimum of side effects should not be too hard to find. But there is one absolute rule here: *do not discontinue any medication without consulting your doctor.* As beneficial as these drugs are, they can cause trouble if stopped suddenly.

□ 9 □

Diet

In former times my idea of a perfect day would have been a breakfast of poached eggs on corned beef hash; a two-hour museum visit followed by a lunch of, say, a nice cheese omelet; watching a baseball game in the afternoon followed by a nap, then a few drinks before a dinner of, say, pasta Alfredo or carbonara, a large rare steak, creamed spinach, Caesar salad; generous pieces of several fine cheeses after dessert (I wasn't too particular about desserts). Now the ideal day starts with cereal and 1% milk; a morning of fishing along a certain spring creek; a large salad with an excellent tomato for lunch; eighteen holes of golf in the afternoon followed by two hours in the evening back along that stream; a dinner of grilled chicken or fish, grilled or steamed vegetables, pasta with garlic and olive oil, and a fresh peach for dessert. The second gives me as much pleasure as the first once did, probably more. Do you know what the real difference between these two is, without being melodramatic? Death and Life. Illness and Health. Then and Now.

There seems to be no end of low-fat diets and guides published for the heart patient; you are now part of a very large and competitive market! Some of them are unofficial and some have the blessing of one authority or another in the form of an "introduction." I certainly have no doubt that these are all well intended and if you follow most of them closely, you probably have nothing to fear beyond being bored to death. My own transition has gone like this:

Pasta Alfredo. Pasta carbonara.
Fried chicken with mashed potatoes and gravy.
Roast beef with mashed potatoes and gravy.
Scalloped potatoes.
Pork roast; ham; pork chops.

Emmenthaler, chèvre, Brie, Brie de Meaux, Chester, Cheshire, Cheddar, Camembert, Caerphilly, Cantal, Isigny, Lancashire, Livarot; Tomme de Cantal, Mignon, Münster, provolone, Gruyère, bleu cheese, Gorgonzola, mozzarella, Gervais, Neufchâtel, Pont L'Evêque, Roquefort.

Butter.

Corned beef hash with two poached eggs.
Spareribs.
Barbecued ribs, country ribs
Deviled beef ribs.

Scrambled eggs, fried eggs, bacon, ham and sausage; hot rolls and butter.

Pâté—any kind of pâté; sweetbreads; kidneys.

A bagel with cream cheese; a cream cheese and olive sandwich; a ham and cheese sandwich.

Cream of mushroom soup, cream of anything soup; cream, cream sauces; quiche.

Pastrami, corned beef, French fried potatoes.

Those lovely sausage dinners—German wursts with

sauerkraut, Italian sausages with peppers.

Rib roast and Yorkshire pudding.

I loved them all.

R.I.P.

Greetings!

Lemon sole, gray sole, rex sole, Dover sole, any sole; Monkfish, codfish, swordfish, wolffish. Tuna fish.

Red snapper.
Mutton snapper, lane snapper, cubera snapper, mangrove snapper, gray snapper.
Halibut.

Vegetables: boiled, steamed, roasted, grilled, raw.
Asparagus; spinach. Zucchini, chayote, broccoli, broccoli rabe, salsify, artichokes, Jerusalem artichokes, arugula; peapods (what the English call mangetout).

Green beans. Peas. Squashes of all sorts and sizes.
Sweet corn.

Tomatoes—real tomatoes, August, September, and October tomatoes; in a lucky year early November tomatoes.
Not January tomatoes, but if you were clever, fresh tomato sauce in January or February.

Basil, thyme, sage, rosemary, savory.
Garlic. A bissel gahlic. What I once read in a recipe printed in an Omaha newspaper: a soup can of garlic.

Salmon—poached salmon, broiled salmon, smoked salmon, pickled salmon, salmon loaf, salmon croquettes, grilled salmon.

Sashimi—tuna, tuna belly (*toro*), fluke, shrimp, octopus, mackerel, urchin, yellowtail. Ahh.

Pastapastapastapasta. Salad—lots of salad.

Finish your greens.

I am not going to offer you a collection of recipes and menus but I do have a strong recommendation in terms of a new (or it was for me) philosophy or approach to food. As anyone who knows me will attest, except for my family and fishing, I love good food *more than anything else on earth*, and I approached these changes with more than a little trepidation. (A few days before I left the hospital, a stunningly attractive woman came to see me and introduced herself as the specialist dietician. I was much charmed by her presence, but almost threw her out of my room as she unfolded the details of my proposed diet. Thinking I would never eat well again was the worst part of that whole hospital stay).

To my surprise, I later found out for myself that a healthy diet does not necessarily mean a boring one. In fact—and you must trust me on this one—it can be more interesting than before because of the increased importance of planning, the greater need for imagination, and the reliance on ingredients with flavor instead of richness. Unless you have no interest in food and are content to eat the same thing most of the time, *this is extremely important* ✳ *since you must change your habits from the very foundations*. If you do not adopt new rules, you will be prone to cutting the corners, first occasionally and soon frequently. Take advantage of your present resolve and you will find that your very tastes and needs will change before you know it. Soon, unhealthy food won't even *taste* good.

Here are a few things I did.

Do you recall the popular image of a horse-drawn sleigh plunging over the Russian snowscape, with various, uh, contents being thrown to the pursuing wolves in order to both (temporarily) mollify them and lighten the load for increased speed? Think of your former regular diet as this sleigh and that you must jettison elements until you can be seen to be pulling away from the wolves of heart disease—and keeping a good distance ahead. Bear in mind that the cholesterol we are discussing is the LDL, the potentially harmful one, and it is found only in animal fats.

First of all, there are a few food types that are so supercharged with cholesterol that they must be abandoned altogether—that's it, finished, good-bye, *finito*, *adios*: liver, kidneys, sweetbreads, brains, and all those other innards known as offal, as well as the foods in which it is hidden, such as liverwurst and pâté. Just forget they exist, now and forever. They'll kill you.

Next come the foods that are quite high in cholesterol: eggs, butter, cream, cheese, ice cream. My basic rule with these is *never when selection is under my control*. I say no to these things at a restaurant or at home—even with a Swedish wife!—but yes, in moderation, when a guest. What this means is that I will eat, within reason, what I am served in someone else's home; it does *not* mean that I have the freedom of the cheese platter or that I am at liberty to slather butter over every roll in sight. Being a guest is one thing, but that status is not to be used as an excuse for going bananas. I am reminded of a friend's father whose doctor told him to limit his drinks to one a week; he found a forty-ounce glass for his whisky and filled (and emptied) it each Friday evening, regular as clockwork. I'm sure he had not drunk that much before the limitations were imposed. However, guest status does not alter the above "offal rule."

It was not easy, but I cut eggs from my diet altogether. Eggs contain about 250 milligrams of cholesterol *each*, slightly less than your target limit (of 300 milligrams) for *an entire day*. I will confess here, for the first time in public, to having consumed two eggs at my wedding breakfast *and* one during my wedding trip. The latter was under the "guest status provision" enumerated above and was the finest egg I ever et. I'll tell you about it sometime. The various egg substitutes such as Egg Beaters, however, are altogether adequate for many purposes, especially in a savory omelet of some sort.

Then went cream in all forms, whipped, iced, in sauces, hidden in rich desserts. This, too, was not easily abandoned, since using it with some butter and Parmesan cheese and *almost anything* else makes a superb and quickly and easily prepared pasta dish. My son and I ate it often. A few tablespoons of heavy cream when added to reduced meat or fish cooking juices and reduced a bit further makes an excellent sauce. Potatoes mashed with cream (and butter) are heaven. And so on. A similar ban is imposed on butter, and for the few times when it is essential, a product called I Can't Believe It's Not Butter is highly recommended. A caution, though: just because it is not butter does not mean it is not fat. All these products— and I'm sure the other butter substitutes are delicious, too—are various kinds of fat, and your intake of them must be severely limited. This suggestion of abstemiousness has been reinforced recently with the publication of research on substances called trans fatty acids, which are formed when liquid vegetable and grain oils are made into solids, a process called hydrogenation. Trans fatty acids have been shown to increase LDL and decrease HDL cholesterol as much as saturated (animal) fats do; those who turned to margarine as a "safe" substitute for butter must continue the search.

The basic problem with the American diet, the one most of us were raised on, is that it is simply too high in fat, and most of the fat we have eaten all these years not only has no nutritional value but has been and is actually harmful. Unfortunately, we have acquired a taste for it since it has such a wonderful flavor (in the form of cheese) and enriches other flavors (such as in meat). Fats also have other "advantages": by slowing the excretion of gastric juices they prolong the digestive process, thus making us feel satisfied and "full" longer; since they take long to digest, we are less likely to have hunger pangs between meals. An obvious solution to this is to eat more frequent and smaller meals. And when that theory was put oto a scientific test it produced an unexpected dividend: the *same* number of calories consumed in seventeen snacks instead of three meals was found to lower LDL cholesterol by 14 percent, a significant amount, and with that a consequent reduction in heart disease risk. But the three-meal-a-day habit would be hard to break and for many of us giving up dinner would be unthinkable.

While on the subject of fat, we need to look at it briefly and *commit it to memory*, since the kinds and amounts of fat we consume are more important than the cholesterol issue. Without going too far into their chemistry, fats are divided into three types of fatty acids: saturated, monounsaturated, and polyunsaturated. If there is no room on the fat molecule for additional atoms of hydrogen, it is said to be saturated; if there is room for two hydrogen atoms, it is monounsaturated; and if it can take four or more it is called polyunsaturated. To be more specific:

Saturated fats are those from animals and the three "tropical" oils: coconut, palm kernel, and palm. As intake of these fats increases, so do levels of total cholesterol and particularly LDL cholesterol, and with them heart disease risk. These fats are to be avoided.

Monounsaturated fats include oils made oil from canola (rape or mustard) seed, olives and, to a lesser extent, peanuts; liquid and stick margarines; hydrogenated vegetable shortening. These probably have the edge in reducing the blood level of the LDL or harmful cholesterol and also generate a kind of cholesterol resistant to free radicals. They are our "fats of choice."

Polyunsaturated fats include oils made from corn, cottonseed, safflower, sesame seed, and sunflower; most tub margarines. These are believed to help lower total blood cholesterol *but* with them the "good" HDL cholesterol, and are also susceptible to free radicals, the very reactive compounds that are the likely cause of plaque development and growth. These fats are to be eaten in moderation.

A logical question would be: Which is the most dangerous fat? The answer is: the fat around your middle.

In case you are beginning to feel you should avoid all dietary fats, here's one you could probably use a lot more of: EPA is short for eicosapentaenoic acid and is a type of polyunsaturated fat found in fish oil. It is one of several fats called Omega-3 fatty acids; they have been found to offer a large number of benefits, such as a decrease in cholesterol and triglyceride levels in the blood; a reduction of blood platelet clumping; and suppression of the production of a substance called thromboxane, which damages arterial walls.

Milk is fairly straightforward: whole milk has about 35 milligrams of cholesterol per cup, low-fat milk a little more than half that, and skim milk only 5 milligrams. If you have a half cup on your morning cereal it probably does not matter much between low-fat and skim, but if you actually drink the stuff, skim is absolutely essential. As for ice cream, I had no difficulty giving it up since I was never all that keen on it to begin with, but I can understand how it could be a problem. Ice cream is butterfat, pure and simple, and is, or can be, murderous to a heart diet. I am informed that frozen yogurt can be an excellent substitute. A word to the wise is sufficient.

I feel about cheese the way others may feel about ice cream, and it remains a real temptation. I allow myself a spoonful or two of grated Parmesan on appropriate pastas but otherwise do not eat it. I don't know about so-called low-fat cheeses but have my doubts; after all, isn't cheese milk fat by definition? Anyway, cool it in the cheese department.

Which brings us to meat. Ah yes, meat. Most of us were raised on red meat, and many have not abandoned it yet. Here's a good time to try to do just that. It is essential to remember that meat is the major dietary source of saturated fat, which promotes the development and growth of atherosclerosis. Except for steak and lamb four or five times a year, I make every effort to put meat in the Only as a Guest Category (and am then secretly disappointed when I'm not served it). This means shunning beef, lamb, ham, pork, in all their varieties, and *especially* sausages, hot dogs, and all those other lovely prepared meats.

There *may* become an exception to this: a newly developed crossbreed of Belgian Blue and Holstein that produces beef with a cholesterol level more than 10 percent below that of chicken breast. I have not tried it yet, but however good it may be, it will not become a regular

Fat Content of Meats, Poultry, Fish, and Other Protein Sources, 3-Ounce Portions

	Total Fat (g)	Saturated Fat (g)	Calories	Cholesterol (mg)
RED MEAT				
Veal top round (roasted)	2.9	1.0	127	88
Pork tenderloin (roasted)	4.1	1.4	133	67
Beef top round (broiled)	4.2	1.4	153	71
Beef eye of round (roasted)	4.2	1.5	143	59
Pork sirloin chop, boneless (broiled)	5.7	1.5	156	78
Pork loin roast, boneless (roasted)	6.4	2.4	160	66
Lamb leg (roasted)	6.6	2.3	162	78
Pork loin chop, bone in (broiled)	6.9	2.5	165	70
Beef tenderloin (broiled)	8.5	3.2	179	71
Frankfurter, beef and pork (boiled)	24.8	9.1	272	42
Pork sausage, country-style (cooked)	26.5	9.2	314	71
POULTRY				
Turkey breast, skinless (roasted)	2.7	0.9	133	59
Chicken breast, skinless (roasted)	3.0	0.9	140	72
Turkey thigh, skinless (roasted)	6.1	2.1	159	72
Chicken thigh, skinless (roasted)	9.3	2.6	178	81
Chicken breast, skin on (fried)	11.2	3.0	221	72
Duck, skin on (roasted)	24.1	8.2	286	71
FISH AND SEAFOOD				
Lobster meat (cooked)	0.5	<0.1	83	61
Scallops, bay or sea (raw)	0.6	<0.1	75	28
Cod (broiled)	0.7	0.1	89	47
Shrimp (moist heat cooked)	0.9	0.2	84	166
Flounder (broiled)	1.3	0.3	99	58
Crab, Alaska king (steamed)	1.3	0.1	82	45
Oysters (eastern, raw)	2.1	0.5	59	47
Tuna, white (canned in water)	2.1	0.6	116	36
Trout, rainbow (broiled)	3.7	0.7	128	62
Tuna, light (canned in oil)	7.0	1.3	168	15
Salmon, sockeye (broiled)	9.3	1.6	184	74
OTHER				
Tofu/bean cured	4.1	0.6	65	0
Eggs (hard-boiled)	9.5	2.8	134	466

	Total Fat (g)	Saturated Fat (g)	Calories	Cholesterol (mg)
American cheese food (pasteurized process)	20.9	13.1	279	54
Cheddar cheese	28.2	17.9	343	89
Peanuts (roasted in shell)	41.4	7.3	495	0
Peanut butter	43.5	7.2	502	0

OK NO! →

Sources: United States Department of Agriculure, *Composition of Foods*, Handbooks 8-1, 8-5, 8-7, 8-10, 8-12, 8-13, 8-15, 8-16, 8-17; HVH-CWRI Nutrient Data Base, reprinted in Ensminger et al., *Food for Health*, Pegus Press, 1986.
[Reprinted from the March 1991 issue of the *Harvard Health Letter*, © 1991, President and Fellows of Harvard College.]

item on our menu: it is very expensive—depending on the cut, up to twenty-five dollars a pound! (Eleventh-hour note: I tried it and it was *excellent*. But it was still very expensive.)

If I have failed to persuade you to give up meat entirely, then at least have small (three to four ounces) portions of the leaner cuts of beef, such as round steak, instead of rib roast and porterhouse steaks. The new approach to breeding pigs has produced leaner meat, too.

There are many charts and guidelines available on this subject. The one above is particularly good.

"What is left to eat?" you might be asking forlornly at this point. Actually, a great deal remains to us, and when prepared with care and imagination it will seem that the choices are greater than before. First of all, there is fish. Some parts of the country have very little of it to offer, it is true, and in other parts it is very expensive. But good fish is becoming more widely available as the demand increases and as air freight becomes less costly. Soon a good variety of fresh deep-water ocean fish will be available across the country at a reasonable cost—that is, if the greedy fishing countries leave anything behind. Studies have shown that eating fish at least twice a week protects the heart from developing abnormal and often fatal rhythms (arrhythmias) and seems to abort the development of lesions on the arterial walls. As important for our purposes, fish is delicious. If you have not cooked fish before, you are in for a great treat: it is very versatile, absorbing other flavors easily; it cooks very quickly; and with most cuts there is no waste. If you are one of those with a phobia about small bones, just buy filets and run your fingers over them before cooking. *There is nothing better for you than fresh fish.* The reason for this is that the oil in fish contains two substances called Omega-3 fatty acids, which have been shown both to lower the levels of triglycerides in the blood and to reduce the likelihood of heart attacks and stroke by inhibiting clotting.

Because it is high in cholesterol, seafood—shrimp, lobster, crabs, and shellfish (oysters, clams, and mussels)—has long been a question mark for many people. I don't see how I could live without it. Dr. William Castelli, the director of the Framingham Heart Study, the oldest, largest, and most thorough study of heart disease, said on this subject: "If you can't be a vegetarian, then eat a vegetarian from the sea—namely, oysters, clams, mussels, and scallops. And, no, I don't think you have to be concerned about lobster or shrimp. You can have them all." That's straight from the horse's mouth and good enough for me.

Chicken and turkey, of course, are widely available and reliable. It's difficult to imagine anything you can't do with either; ground turkey, for instance, replaces ground beef in *any* dish but a hamburger, and I defy anyone to tell them apart in casseroles, meatloaf, sauce for pasta, and so on. Of course poultry is also less costly and more versatile than meat.

And the leaner cuts of veal are available, too, to be eaten in moderation. Like lobster, good veal is quite expensive, but there is little waste, if any, depending on the cut, and it, too, is versatile. We reserve it for special occasions and enjoy it very much.

Many Americans see green vegetables as something they must eat with a complete dinner but do so only out of obligation. Well, I'm here to tell you that greens *can* be absolutely wonderful. If you don't already know how to cook them properly, it's time to learn because the contrast between good and awful is amazing. Spinach steamed until it barely wilts, drained, and then quickly sautéed in a small amount of olive oil with a little garlic is ambrosia; the same vegetable overcooked is disgusting. Despite George Bush's childish and defiant pronouncements on the subject, broccoli is an excellent vegetable and recently was shown to contain a powerful anticancer agent. I peel then steam it until a knife just pierces it, then serve it as is or sautéed in olive oil with garlic or sesame seeds. Recently, many vegetables—broccoli rabe, zucchini squash, peapods, and asparagus, to name some of them— are not only more widely available but also have a much longer season. Take advantage of them! Not long ago, in the West and Midwest, iceberg lettuce was the only leafy green easily found; now even small stores in obscure places carry an amazing array of greens. Thank heavens!

And here's a tip for the end of the meal: a Dutch study showed that boiled coffee—as opposed to filtered or drip—raised levels of LDL cholesterol dramatically, so avoid this method of preparation. In New York they would say "Go figure."

Obviously I could go on and on. There are many books on the market that offer Heart Smart diets, and there is an excellent magazine, *Eating Well*, devoted to the subject. I'll just urge two more categories of food that may not have occurred to you. Pasta is widely available in a great variety of forms. As the Italians have known for centuries (and learned from the Chinese via Marco Polo), few foods are more versatile or more healthy. And here's a little reward for having read this far: there's a type of pasta called orzo (or sometimes riso) that is the size and shape of rice. Unlike most pasta, it is hard to overcook. It is excellent hot—plain or with a little grated Parmesan cheese or with finely chopped vegetables—and also makes excellent salads, mixed with chopped peppers or other vegetables or meat or chicken or shrimp or or or. One could literally write a cookbook devoted exclusively to orzo. Of course like other pastas, the dried form lasts on your shelf forever.

One more tip before we proceed to the subject of exercise. Dried beans. Yes, you heard me, dried beans. In many cooks' hands this versatile and extremely healthy food is a horror, but when you learn to cook beans correctly you find them to be delicious. They are also available in a great variety of types and tastes. The secret is to soak them for a day or so, changing the water whenever you get around to it but at least several times. Out with the water will go most if not all of the elements that produce gas or other gastric upset. Then boil them slowly with richly flavored things like broth or smoked meat and/or herbs—there's plenty of room to experiment. Black beans, simmered with a ham bone, an onion stuck with a few cloves, a bay leaf or two, and some thyme, then served with rice and some chopped onion is out of this world! Red beans cooked with... well, I think I've made the point. Give beans a shot.

❑ 10 ❑

Exercise

In the good old days—at least my good old days—there was no time reserved for voluntary exercise. Even though I was somewhat of an athlete as a youth, smoking did a pretty good job of squashing any physical activity. I preferred sitting, reading, and smoking to a trip to the gym *any* day. Nowadays, my typical routine includes at least a full hour at the gym, plus walking whenever possible, plus plus plus. I am still far from where I would like to be in the exercise department, but I am moving in the right direction.

In addition to increasing your own sense of well-being, exercise strengthens the heart muscle because exertion requires the heart to pump more blood; a stronger heart pumps more blood each beat and therefore does not need to beat as often. Exercise reduces stress because it lowers the level of hormones that speed up the heart rate and increase blood pressure. And it can be fun!

It is important to differentiate between the two types of exercise, *dynamic* or *aerobic* or *cardiovascular (C.V.)*, versus *static*. Your heart is a muscle, and like other muscles it performs more efficiently if it is strong and healthy. Dynamic exercise—jogging, bicycling, swimming, jumping rope—calls on the heart and circulatory system to do more work to deliver oxygen to the body's tissues to provide the energy being used. The idea is to increase the heart rate, the number of beats per minute, and to sustain that higher level for a reasonable period of time. In time, and you'll be surprised how quickly, your heart will function more efficiently at a lower level for a longer time, and you will be very much the better for it.

Static exercise—lifting weights, chopping wood, shoveling snow, using Nautilus or Eagle machines—is sporadic and therefore does not keep your heart rate sustained at a higher level for any beneficial length of time. It *can* be dangerous if unprepared for, as it could put an unexpected strain on the heart. It is, however, at least for me, more fun, so by all means include some of it in your program. It also offers more visible rewards, such as larger and better developed muscles.

Maintaining interest and enjoyment is essential to the life and success of your exercise regimen. If it is too boring or unpleasant you will find ways to avoid it. Find a gym that is clean, bright, and well kept, where both sexes work out and where the average age is less than yours. The more pleasant the atmosphere, the more you will look forward to going there or at least the less you will *avoid* going there. A hint: if at all possible, get a trainer and work with him or her two or preferably three times a week. This makes the time go more quickly and efficiently; you will have a more effective regimen; and there will be someone there in the unlikely event of a problem (early in my post-operative exercise career I had an arrhythmia or fibrillation that was caught while working out with a trainer). Your appointment with your trainer will get you moving when excuses present themselves—which they can do very conveniently. Most important, exercising is much more fun if done with the right person. I owe my trainer, Milton Swaby, much of the credit for my present health, but if you quote this to him I will deny every word. We have a good time together and a lot of laughs. That's important, because effective exercise is boring.

From time to time you read about someone suffering a fatal heart attack during strenuous exercise such as shoveling snow or chopping wood, and it is true that many fatal heart attacks occur in such circumstances. It is tempting to conclude that such exercise is harmful and to avoid it. There is a hidden truth here, though, and that is that these heart attacks occur among the proverbial couch potatoes who are not accustomed to exercise. Studies show that sedentary people are *a hundred times* more likely to have a heart attack in such circumstances than those in reasonably good shape (and age is no barrier to staying in shape). You have probably also noted that people in shape seem to have fewer illnesses and ailments, major or minor.

Most authorities on this subject seem to agree that a healthy level of exercise expends two thousand calories per week. They recommend steady, not strenuous, exercise. Don't try to fulfill your weekly goal in one afternoon!

Your choice of exercise method is of particular importance, since if it becomes *too* boring you will find excuses to avoid it. Here are some particular recommendations:

Bicycling. This is a fine form of exercise because it requires steady exertion and you must be at least reasonably alert (or you'll fall off). You must, however, live in or near appropriate terrain: you want an area that is fairly flat, so you can avoid the strain of hills, and reasonably traffic-free so that you don't get hit. A stationary bicycle is an excellent indoor alternative, but be sure to use it around other people, in front of a television, or listening to music. Otherwise, since their use is so boring, they will likely be soon abandoned.

Rowing machines. It may be because I enjoyed rowing boats as a child that I get pleasure out of working these machines, even though, as with the stationary bicycle, a lot of effort gets you absolutely nowhere. There are now machines with computerized races and graphic images of the "places" where you are rowing, and they are entertaining. Such machines are quite expensive and generally found only in up-market sports clubs.

Stair or step machines. Very popular in almost any gym you might enter, but I think they're the pits. You can't read on them and you'll get a crick in the neck if you try to watch television. At sixteen steps per flight, I think I have climbed about a million flights of stairs on these machines and I hope I never see one again. But many people love them, and maybe you will, too.

Swimming. Perhaps this is the ideal exercise for you because it puts the least strain on your body. Like walking, there are no sudden stops, starts, or strains, and you are more likely to feel refreshed and energized at the end than exhausted. It is particularly beneficial for those who are either overweight or unsteady because of the buoyancy of the water. Swimming contributes greatly to good body tone, something you will be keenly aware of as you begin to achieve it. More and more health clubs and towns have indoor pools and they are well worth seeking out.

Treadmill. This puts minimum strain on your body, is under your control (you can increase speed and angle at will), and is fairly safe, although falling is not unusual. You can probably get as much good exercise in a short period of time on a treadmill as with any form of working out; but be sure to have music, reading, or television available because using a treadmill is boring.

Burning Calories

Activity	Calories/Hour	Hours/Week
Walking (2 mph)	290	7
Fast Walking (4.5 mph)	360	5½
Jogging (5.5 mph)	750	3
Running (10 mph)	1,000	2
Swimming (50 yds./min)	760	3
Bicycling (13 mph)	840	2½
Aerobic dancing	390	5½
Stair climbing	45 per 100 steps	
Horseback riding	275	8
Roller skating	400	5
Skiing (Cross-country)	800	2½
Skiing (Downhill)	690	3
Squash	690	3
Tennis (Doubles)	360	6
Tennis (Singles)	480	4½
Shooting pool	150	13¼
Gardening	300	6¾

Walking. This is an excellent form of exercise because you can do it almost anywhere and in many different conditions; there is often so much stimulation that you forget you are exercising (for example, walking in an unfamiliar city). You can do it outdoors or in (malls around the country seem to be filled with people exercising), and unless you require special shoes, there is no cost!

The table opposite will tell you how much you should do of what. While the actual number of calories expended varies according to several factors, the information contained in the table generally holds true.

The best plan is to combine a number of these activities that will burn at least two thousand calories. Many of us used to think that seeking fitness was a waste of time, but now one can safely say it is essential to good health. By the way, I did not make up these numbers: I took them from the January/February 1988 issue of *Hippocrates* magazine. Similar figures were published in an article by William Stockton in the *New York Times* of November 16, 1987, among other places.

Any exercise is better than no exercise!

A dividend from following a fitness plan may well be an increased likelihood of collateralization, whereby small blood vessels develop on the heart near and around the blockages, providing an increased blood supply to the heart. You might think of them as natural bypasses, and for them there is no risk and no charge.

□ 11 □

Alcohol

The consumption of alcohol, which for some reason we just call *drinking*, may be as important to understand in terms of heart health as hypertension, diet, and exercise, since it, too, is within your control.

First of all, drinking does not cause heart disease; it is not even one of the direct contributing factors, major or minor, like high blood fats or smoking. Its indirect effect, however, can be very great indeed. As much as diet and exercise, and maybe even more, alcohol consumption has a considerable influence on your overall health and general fitness: the more healthy and fit you are, the greater is your ability to withstand heart disease. Immoderate drinking will be more harmful to your general health than almost anything else.

For some people, drinking in moderation may be a part of good general health; it helps many to relax, thus contributing to lower blood pressure, and it helps many to digest food. What is "moderate"? The U.S. Surgeon General's *Report on Nutrition and Health* (1988) recommended no more than two drinks per day, so we'll go along with that, as did the Harvard study described in this chapter. This means two 12-ounce beers; two 5-ounce glasses of wine; two mixed drinks containing 1½ ounces of liquor each; or a combination of these. Of course this varies according to your own metabolism and comfort—and don't start drinking alcohol as a preventive measure, as there are many for whom it is harmful. But on the other hand, don't give up that pleasurable glass of wine with dinner because you heard somewhere that it would give you a heart attack (it won't). Most important of all, consult your doctor and be honest about how much you really drink. Between the two of you, a plan for optimum health and comfort should be easily established.

It is alleged—by Inserm, the French equivalent of the National Institute of Health—that French red wine has a flushing effect on arterial walls. A report that received much attention at the end of 1991 suggested that a moderate intake of wine was the reason for a 40 percent lower incidence of coronary heart disease in France than in the United States, despite a diet that includes foods very high in fat (foie gras, cheese, cream, eggs, and so on). Scientists generally agree that *moderate alcohol consumption can reduce the risk of heart disease.*

A study at Harvard of what is called the French Paradox showed that two drinks a day for six weeks (in a study group of adults who had not consumed alcohol before) increased HDL cholesterol by 17 *percent* in that brief period. Even more startling are the results of a recently published study: the alcohol consumption of 6,051 men and 7,234 women between the ages of thirty and seventy in Copenhagen, Denmark, was carefully monitored over a period of twelve years, from 1976 to 1988. In the words of the report, "the risk of dying decreased with an increasing intake of wine—from a relative risk of 1.00 for the subjects who never drank wine to 0.51 for those who drank three to five glasses a day. Intake of neither beer nor spirits, however, was associated with reduced risk. For spirits intake the relative risk of dying increased from 1.00 for those who never drank to 1.34 for those with an intake of three to five drinks a day. The effects of the three types of alcoholic drinks seemed to be independent of each other, and no significant interactions existed with sex, age, education, income, smoking, or body mass index. Wine drinking showed the same relation to risk of death from cardiovascular and cerebrovascular disease as to risk of death from all causes." Indeed, the Copenhagen study showed an almost direct relationship between wine consumption and reduction in mortality risk.

Moderate alcohol consumption, as stated above, has been shown to reduce the risk of heart attack, and a recent study in the Netherlands has shown why. Within an hour of ingesting alcohol, and lasting twelve hours or more, the body's mechanism for dissolving blood clots is unusually and measurably active. That means the risk of heart attack is lowered not only *during* this period (since many heart attacks are caused by the encounter of a moving blood clot with an arterial wall obstruction, thus slowing or stopping normal blood flow), but *after* as well, since potentially dangerous clots are either dissolved or reduced to a less threatening size.

To return briefly to the "French Paradox": the chemical that decreases the level of LDL cholesterol in blood— resveratrol—was isolated by Dr. Leroy Creasy, a fruit cultivation specialist at the New York State College of Agriculture and Life Sciences at Cornell University. Resveratrol is found in all products of the grape, especially in the juice of Concord grapes. Tests in rats demonstrated that resveratrol reduces levels of cholesterol *and* the clumping of blood cells that leads to atherosclerosis and heart attacks. So take heart! The same level of protection is available to those who do not drink wine, since grape juice contains as much resveratrol as wine.

There are two more things to bear in mind, either or both of which may apply to you: If you take a prescribed medication, it is essential that you consult with your physician *with full disclosure of your drinking habits,* since some medications are diminished in strength or rendered ineffective by alcohol. And if weight is a problem, remember that alcohol contains no significant nutrients and is high in calories. Nothing will put—or keep—weight on like alcohol. If there is one truth in this book I could change, it would probably be this one, but there you are.

□ 12 □

Medications

First and foremost there is aspirin. Unless you are under doctor's instructions not to do so, put this book down and go take one right now, and every day for the rest of your life (which is likely to be longer as a result). All those with cardiac risk factors should be taking an aspirin a day, and for all those who have undergone heart surgery it is essential to take an aspirin a day. If normal doses of this drug have upset you in the past, you should know that you only need about a quarter of an average tablet each day (the recommended dose is 75 milligrams and a tablet contains 325 milligrams). *This dosage reduces the chances of a heart attack or stroke by 50 percent.*

Heart attacks are usually caused by blood clots being stopped in a coronary artery narrowed by disease. One of the factors involved in blood clotting is the aggregation of particles called platelets, and aspirin inhibits that aggregation by reducing the stickiness of the platelets. This process was discovered and described by the pharmacologist John Vane and was considered to be of such significance that he was awarded the Nobel Prize for Medicine, in 1982. The number of lives that have been saved by this discovery is incalculable.

In a study of heart attack among 22,071 doctors, half were given an aspirin every other day, half were given an imitation—what is called a placebo. After five years, there had been 293 heart attacks in the whole group, of which 23 were fatal; 189 including 18 fatal were from the group that did not take aspirin. The study was stopped, and everybody took the aspirin, one would hope even the researchers.

In January 1994, the *British Medical Journal* devoted fifty pages over three successive issues (itself without precedent) to a detailed report of something called the Antiplatelet Trialists' Collaboration. This combined the results from 300 distinct clinical trials involving more than 140,000 patients to arrive at a single recommendation: after consultation with a physician, everyone who has ever had coronary bypass surgery, a heart attack, angina pectoris, or a stroke should take one-half or one aspirin tablet each day unless there is a reason not to. It is estimated that adherence to this simple rule would prevent more than 200,000 nonfatal strokes and heart attacks each year and about 100,000 fatal ones.

It is to be hoped you won't need nitroglycerin, but not at all unlikely that you will. The chest pain that kicked off this whole adventure may well return, if in a milder and certainly less frightening form, from any of a variety of sources. For this kind of pain, nitroglycerin is the medicine of choice. If you have not made its acquaintance yet, you probably should.

It is available in a number of forms but most commonly in a tiny pill under the brand name Nitrostat. It is taken *sublingually*, which means placed under the tongue to be absorbed and is *not swallowed*! It provides very prompt relief from the pain of angina, and it is probably a good idea to keep some with you all the time. There are two reasons why it might be wise to try Nitrostat if you haven't yet taken any: you will become more confident about the method of taking it, and you will experience its effects so that they may become familiar and not intimidating. You will probably have a brief, slight, headache and a flushed feeling. Some people feel a slight dizziness. Nitroglycerin is a vasodilator, which means it widens or dilates the coronary arteries (and other arteries as well). As you remember, angina is caused by the coronary arteries' inability to supply sufficient blood to the heart, and this chemical increases that supply quickly, making you feel a lot better a lot faster. This is a wonderful drug and we have Alfred Nobel, the donor of the prizes that bear his name, and serendipity to thank for it. In its pure form, nitroglycerin is *very* explosive and *very* unstable. Nobel invented a way to stabilize it, thereby inventing dynamite, and a way to destabilize the dynamite, thereby making it useful.

Nitroglycerin was actually first made by an Italian chemist named Ascanio Sobrero. Aware of its unstable and highly explosive properties, he nevertheless tasted it and found that it was sweet and it left him with a throbbing headache. Reports of this circulated in the scientific community, and tasting nitroglycerin as a kind of scientific lark spread quickly. (It was an age when such things were done lightly.) A young English physician named William Murrell tried it and remembered that another nitrogen compound, amyl nitrate, produced a similar headache but was also known to relieve a specific kind of chest pain that otherwise defied treatment. Murrell had a patient with this affliction for whom he prescribed a weak solution of the new chemical. The patient received immediate relief and took to carrying a vial of it around with him to use as needed. Soon the use of very small amounts of nitroglycerin for angina became widespread.

It was during this time that Alfred Nobel was developing his process of stabilizing nitroglycerin. His invention, dynamite, was probably the most destructive commercial product ever: It changed the course of history. The fortune made from this and other inventions of his was left to a foundation, the income of which was to be used for annual prizes for significant contributions to mankind in five (later increased to six) categories: Physics, Chemistry, Medicine, Peace, and Literature. (Economics was added in 1969.)

Nobel himself suffered from debilitating heart disease. He retired to Paris to complete his will and was only able to do so because of the relief offered by Murrell's discovery. In 1895, Nobel wrote: "It sounds like the irony of fate, that I should be ordered to take nitroglycerin internally."

Nitoglycerin is one of a group of chemicals called nitrates, which mean their molecules contain the element nitrogen; other forms are used in pills, capsules, ointments, patches, and solutions for injections. They are wonderful, wonderful drugs and have made many pain- and worry-ridden lives not only bearable but symptom-free. They are inexpensive and non–habit forming. They are seldom known to have side effects.

After you have fully returned to a normal life—that is to say, once you have changed your patterns of eating, drinking, exercise, and have stopped smoking cigarettes—a few fairly simple medical tests will inform your doctor what adjustments should be made by medication. Your cholesterol level will have plummeted after your surgery (I keep reports from those days to look at secretly and longingly), but may well have crept back up to dangerous levels despite your efforts to maintain a diet. Only you know if you are to blame for higher levels. If you have behaved fairly responsibly, and the numbers are still too high, there is a new family of drugs your doctor may seriously consider.

Lovastatin, sold under the brand name Mevacor (Merck), would seem to be one of the few real "miracle" drugs. By actually inhibiting the production of cholesterol by your liver, Mevacor lowers the level of cholesterol in your blood as much as 18 to 34 percent, depending on the dosage, and lowers the damaging LDL cholesterol 19 to 39 percent without affecting the levels of the beneficial HDL cholesterol. These numbers come from a four-year study by the U.S. Food and Drug Administration, not from my back pocket. About 1 percent of the people in the study showed an increase in liver function, so it is important to monitor your body chemistry. Annual eye tests are also urged, since a small number of people have experienced changes in the lens, which could mean a higher risk of developing cataracts. You'll be having plenty of checkups in the future anyway, so just add these two to the list of possible suspects.

Mevacor has, so far, three descendents: pravastatin, simvastatin, and fluvastatin, whose brand names are Pravachol (Bristol-Myers Squibb), Zocor (Merck), and Lescol (Sandoz), respectively. They are all members of a group of medicines called Hmg-CoA reductase inhibitors, and are called statins for short. They work by blocking an enzyme essential to the body in the manufacture of cholesterol. Pravachol and Zocor are associated with decreased levels of triglycerides as well.

After extensive testing, the Food and Drug Administration allowed the manufacturers of Zocor to use the dramatic term "Life Saving." And so it has proved to be. A study among 4,444 patients in Scandinavia with coronary heart disease and high cholesterol for a median length of 5.4 years showed a reduced risk of heart attack or heart disease–related death of 34 *percent* in patients treated with Zocor as contrasted with a group taking a placebo. Another study showed a reduction of coronary death by 43 *percent*. Dramatic numbers indeed!

Anemia is a common condition following heart surgery. Its symptoms may be disguised by the inevitable fatigue and weakness that result from extensive surgery, but anemia is easily detected in a simple blood test. The standard treatment for it is a medication containing iron and a (temporary!) iron-enriched diet.

As time goes by it is not at all unlikely that symptoms of your disease will recur—let's not forget that the surgery dealt only with the *effects* of the disease, not the disease itself. While we hope you will never again experience angina pectoris, it is wise to be prepared for it and informed about controlling or living with it. There are literally scores of cardiac drugs, and individual reactions to them vary considerably. By working closely with your physician, you will be able to establish a regimen of medication that will increase your comfort, prolong your life, and maintain the quality of your life.

It is likely your medication will be either an ACE inhibitor, a beta-blocker, or a calcium channel-blocker (see the following table for descriptions of drugs). Many of these drugs have disturbing side effects, so at the beginning of drug therapy be attentive to changes in your body and mix and match—under your doctor's guidance—until you find the right drug or combination. The effectiveness of these drugs lies in their ability to slow the activity of the heart. They are depressants and may have a depressing effect on you in other ways, too. I regret to report that they may depress the libido. These effects were denied in a recent report, but I'm here to tell you they do exist, if perhaps rarely.

Some Oral Antihypertensive Drugs

Drug	Daily adult dosage	Frequent or severe adverse effects
DIURETICS		
THIAZIDE-TYPE	(Usually once daily)	Hyperuricemia; hypokalemia; hypomagnesemia;
Bendroflumethiazide (*Naturetin*)	2.5-5 mg	hyperglycemia; hyponatremia; hypercalcemia; hyper-
Benzthiazide (*Exna*, others)	12.5-50 mg	cholesterolemia; hypertriglyceridemia; pan-
Chlorothiazide (*Diuril*, others)	125-500 mg	creatitis; rashes and other allergic reactions; weakness;
Cyclothiazide (*Anhydron*)	1-2 mg	sexual dysfunction
Hydrochlorothiazide (*Esidrix*, others)	12.5-50 mg	
Hydroflumethiazide (*Saluron*, others)	12.5-50 mg	
Methyclothiazide (*Enduron*, others)	2.5-5 mg	
Polythiazide (*Renese*)	1-4 mg	
Trichlormethiazide (*Naqua*, others)	1-4 mg	
Chlorthalidone (*Hygroton*, others)	12.5-50 mg	
Indapamide (*Lozol*)	2.5-5 mg	
Metolazone (*Zaroxolyn*, *Mykrox*)	1.25-5 mg Zaroxolyn 0.5-1 mg Mydrox	
Quinethazone (*Hydromox*)	25-100 mg	
LOOP DIURETICS		
Bumetanide (*Bumex*)	0.5-5 mg in 1 or 2 doses	Dehydration; circulatory collapse; hypokalemia;
Ethacrynic acid (*Edecrin*)	12.5-100 mg in 1 or 2 doses	hyponatremia; hypomagnesemia; hypocalcemia;
Furosemide (*Lasix*, others)	20-320 mg in 1 or 2 doses	hyperglycemia; metabolic alkalosis; hyperuricemia; blood dyscrasias; rashes; lipid changes as with thiazide-type diuretics
POTASSIUM-SPARING		
Amiloride (*Midamor*, others)	5-10 mg in 1 or 2 doses	Hyperkalemia; GI disturbances; rash; headache

Drug	Daily adult dosage	Frequent or severe adverse effects
Spironolactone *(Aldactone,* others)	25-100 mg in 1 or 2 doses	Hyperkalemia; hyponatremia; mastodynia; gynecomastia; agranulocytosis; menstrual abnormalities; GI disturbances; rash
Trimterene *(Dyrenium)*	50-150 mg in 1 or 2 doses	Hyperkalemia; GI disturbances; nephrolithiasis

COMBINATIONS

Aldactazide (hydrochlorothiazide 25 or 50 mg, spironolactone 25 or 50 mg)	1 tablet in 1 dose	
Dyazide (hydrochlorothiazide 25 mg, triamterene 50 mg)	1-2 capsules in 1 dose	Similar to individual components
Maxzide (hydrochlorothiazide 25-50 mg, triamterene 37.5 or 75 mg)	1 tablet in 1 dose	
Moduretic (hydrochlorothiazide 50 mg, amiloride 5 mg)	1/2-1 tablet in 1 dose	

ACE (ANGIOTENSIN-CONVERTING ENZYME) INHIBITORS

Benazepril *(Lotensin)*	10-40 mg in 1 or 2 doses	Cough; hypotension, particularly with a diuretic or volume depletion; loss of taste with anorexia; rash; acute renal failure with bilateral renal artery stenosis or stenosis of the artery to a solitary kidney; cholestatic jaundice; pancreatitis; angioedema; hyperkalemia if also taking potassium supplements or potassium-sparing diuretics; blood dyscrasias and renal damage rare except in patients with renal dysfunction; may increase fetal mortality and should not be used during second and third trimesters of pregnancy; may decrease excretion of lithium
Captopril *(Capoten)*	12.5-150 mg in 2 or 3 doses	
Enalapril *(Vasotec)*	2.5-40 mg in 1 or 2 doses	
Fosinopril *(Monopril)*	10-40 mg in 1 or 2 doses	
Lisinopril *(Prinivil, Zestril)*	5-40 mg in 1 dose	
Quinapril *(Accupril)*	5-80 mg in 1 or 2 doses	
Ramipril *(Altace)*	1.25-20 mg in 1 or 2 doses	

Drug	Daily adult dosage	Frequent or severe adverse effects
ALPHA-ADRENERGIC BLOCKERS		
Prazosin (*Minipress*, others)	First day: 1 mg at bedtime Maintenance: 1-20 mg in 2 doses	Syncope with first dose; dizziness and vertigo; palpitations; fluid retention; headache; drowsiness; weakness; anticholinergic effects; priapism; urinary incontinence
Terazosin (*Hytrin*)	First day: 1 mg at bedtime Maintenance: 1-20 mg in 1 dose	Similar to prazosin
Doxazosin (*Cadura*)	First day: 1 mg at bedtime Maintenance: 1-16 mg in 1 dose	Similar to prazosin, but with less hypotension after first dose
PERIPHERAL ADRENERGIC NEURON ANTAGONISTS		
Guanethidine (*Ismelin*)	10-100 mg in 1 dose	Orthostatic hypotension; exercise hypotension; diarrhea; may aggravae bronchial asthma; bradycardia; sodium and water retention; retrograde ejacualtion
Guanadrel (*Hylorel*)	10-75 mg in 2 doses	Similar t oguanethidine, but less diarrhea; aggravation of asthma has not been reported
Reserpine (*Serpasil*, others)	0.05-0.1 mg in 1 dose	Psychic depression; nightmares; nasal stuffiness; drowsiness; GI disturbances; bradycardia
BETA-BLOCKERS		
Atenolol (*Tenormin*, others)	25-100 mg in 1 dose	Fatigue; depression; bradycardia; decreased exercise tolerance; congestive heart failure; aggravate peripheral arterial insufficiency; GI disturbances; bronchospasm; mask symptoms of hypoglycemia; Raynaud's phenomenon; insomnia; vivid dreams or hallucinations; organic grain syndrome; rare blood dyscrasias and other allergic
Betaxolol (*Kerlone*)	5-40 mg in 1 dose	
Metoprolol (*Lopressor, Toprol XL*)	50-200 mg in 1 or 2 doses	
Nadolol (*Corgard*)	20-240 mg in 1 dose	
Propranolol (*Inderal*, others)	40-240 mg in 1 or 2 doses	
Timolol (*Blocadren*)	10-40 mg in 2 doses	

Drug	Daily adult dosage	Frequent or severe adverse effects
		disorders; increased serum triglycerides, decreased HDL cholesterol; generalized pustular psoriasis; transient hearing loss; sudden withdrawal can lead to exacerbation of angina and myocardial infarction
BETA-ADRENERGIC BLOCKING DRUGS WITH ISA		
Acebutolol *(Sectral)*	200-1200 mg in 1 or 2 doses	Similar to other beta-adrenergic blocking drugs, but with less resting bradycardia and lipid changes; acebutolol is cardioselective at low doses and use can be associated with a positive antinuclear antibody test and occasional drug-induced lupus
Carteolol *(Cartrol)*	2.5-10 mg in 1 dose	
Penbutolol *(Lelvatol)*	20-80 mg in 1 dose	
Pindolol *(Visken)*	10-60 mg in 2 doses	
ALPHA-BETA-BLOCKER		
Labetalol *(Trandate, Normodyne)*	200-1200 mg in 1 or 2 doses	Similar to other beta-adrenergic blocking drugs, but has intrinsic sympathomimetic activity and more orthostatic hypotension; fever; hepatotoxicity
CALCIUM-CHANNEL BLOCKERS		
Diltiazem *(Cardizem SR)*	120-360 mg in 2 doses	
(Cardizem CD) *(Dilacor XR)*	120-360 mg in 1 dose	Dizziness; headache; edema; constipation (especially verapamil); AV block; bradycardia; heart failure; gingival hyperplasia
Verapamil (*Calan* and others)	120-480 mg in 2 or 3 doses	
(Calan SR)	120-480 mg in 1 or 2 doses	
(Verelan)	120-480 mg in 1 dose	
DIHYDROPYRIDINES		
Amlodipine *(Norvasc)*	2.5-10 mg in 1 dose	Dizziness; headache; peripheral edema (more than with verapamil); flushing; tachycardia; rash; gingival hyperplasia (nifedipine)
Felodipine *(Plendil)*	5-20 mg in 1 dose	
Isradipine *(DynaCirc)*	5-10 mg in 1 or 2 doses	

Drug	Daily adult dosage	Frequent or severe adverse effects
Nicardipine *(Cardene)*	60-120 mg in 3 doses	
(Cardene SR)	60-120 mg in 2 doses	
Nifedipine *(Procardia XL)*	30-90 mg in 1 dose	

[Reprinted from issue 899, vol. 35, June 25, 1993, of *The Medical Letter on Drugs and Therapeutics* by special permission of the publisher.]

□ 13 □

Reversing Heart Disease

By now you should have a clear idea of what coronary heart disease is, why you developed it, how far it progressed before you became aware of it, how modern science was able to diagnose the extent of its damage and rescue you from the brink of destruction, and the steps you must take to prevent a recurrence of the potentially deadly effects of the disease. I am now going to tell you about a remarkable man who made no discovery or invention, but who took information that was widely known and accepted by the scientific community, and used it to produce a radically new approach to treating coronary heart disease. His proposals initially met with skepticism, but the results are so dramatic as to command our attention, respect, and, indeed, admiration. While the original intent of this program was to avoid coronary bypass surgery *and* prolonged disease management by medication (and it is now too late for you to contemplate it as an alternative), it very probably will work for you if you want to be absolutely sure of avoiding a recurrence of all you have recently endured. For if you have come away with only one lesson, it must be that while the surgery has relieved you of the symptoms of heart disease (or soon will), the disease itself soldiers on, day and night, continuing to wreak destruction and trying to kill you.

The remarkable man I'm talking about is Dean Ornish. He is one of those people whose work is either sworn by or sworn at. Because he does his work in California, and because there is an important spiritual component to what he does, he has been easy to dismiss by some (I have wondered if he would have been received differently had he worked in Delaware, say, or Ohio) but his results speak for themselves.

First of all, we must point out that he is no self-trained seer. He has impeccable academic credentials, having been classically educated (Rice, the University of Texas at Austin, *summa cum laude*; Baylor Medical College) and trained (Massachusetts General Hospital and Harvard). In his second year in medical school he began to look at coronary heart disease, the nation's number-one killer, from various directions and arrived at the conclusion that the disease in its clinical manifestations, that is to say, by the time the patient is aware of being afflicted with it, was the product, after many years, of three factors: diet, exercise (actually lack thereof), and stress. Except for the third factor this was, in fact, accepted medical truth. What was not accepted, and what was perceived as radical, was his postulate that while these factors *produced* the harmful symptoms of heart disease, their *reversal* could undo this damage: that adopting healthy life habits could open clogged arteries and not only increase circulation but also improve general health and a *sense of well-being*. For without the latter, the rest was essentially not even worth the effort.

Ornish's theory, elegant in its simplicity, wanted proving, but because of its unorthodox nature, traditional sources of financial support were closed to him. A few wealthy Texas businessmen, however, were intrigued by the notion that there might be an alternative to the very costly (as you have seen) choices of medication or surgery. They provided the initial funding for the Lifestyle Heart Trial, which was carried out in San Francisco and whose first results were published in 1989.

From an initial pool of patients who had demonstrated symptoms of severe coronary heart disease, forty-eight were chosen with demonstrable (by angiogram) coronary artery occlusion of at least 40 percent and ranging to almost 100 percent. (Patients with severe left, or main, artery disease were excluded.) Twenty-four were put on the standard medical regimen for heart disease: restriction of dietary fat to 30 percent of calories, quitting smoking, and a half hour of aerobic (dynamic) exercise three times a week. This was the control group.

The other half, the test group, had a more strict set of orders: abandon smoking, of course; diet, strictly vegetarian and fat intake only *8 percent* of daily calories: nonfat dairy products and egg whites and *no* animal products of any kind. Alcohol consumption was limited to two ounces a day. In addition to the diet, an hour a day was to be spent practicing stress management techniques: deep relaxation, yoga, stretching, meditation, and special breathing exercises. All were to exercise for an hour three times a week, twice as much as the control group; using pictures of blocked arteries, they learned to visualize their own coronary arteries becoming increasingly more clear; and they met twice a week for four-hour sessions in which they ate, exercised, practiced stress-reducing techniques, discussed their lives and challenges, and provided emotional support for each other.

All the patients in both groups continued being treated by their own physicians, the only change in earlier treatment being a cessation of all cholesterol-lowering medication.

After a year the entire group of forty-eight was to be subjected to blind studies at the Center for Cardiovascular and Imaging Research at the University of Texas Medical School in Houston. The tests were to be as thorough as technology allowed. For various reasons—death not among them—only forty-one were able to go to Houston, twenty-two in the treatment group and nineteen in the control.

Hold on to your hat.

Among the participants in the test group, one had not followed the regimen and the heart disease was worse; three stayed about the same; *eighteen* demonstrated marked improvement, with measurably reduced blockages and increased blood flow to the heart, called coronary flow reserve.

The control group had not fared as well; ten got worse, three stayed the same, six showed modest improvement. As a group, coronary occlusion had increased about 10 percent and coronary flow reserve had decreased significantly.

Dramatic results indeed. And similar ones continue to be achieved. But why bring this up here, after you've already had, or decided on, your surgery? There are three reasons. First of all, to remind you that your surgery is able to deal only with symptoms, and that the underlying disease requires utmost vigilance, now and for the rest of your life; second, to assure you that radical steps of prevention, even at this late stage, are likely to have dramatic results; and third, something I strongly believe in, to emphasize that stress management is the key difference between Dr. Ornish's program and studies of similar groups and the reason for its success.

The Ornish Plan has been criticized in many quarters, but as the man says, you can't argue with success. Of course to a good scientist "stress management" is anathema because both "stress" and its "management" are indefinable and consequently not measurable. But no one can deny that they do exist, and you will ignore them at your peril.

I can do no better than to end with Dean Ornish's own words, as quoted in an interview in the *New York Times*: "Can these comprehensive life-style changes be sustained in larger populations of patients with coronary heart disease? The point of our study was to determine what is true, not what is practicable.

"Heart disease is only a model and a metaphor for what I'm doing and it is certainly not limited to heart disease. It is about trying to help people heal their lives in ways that go beyond illness. The idea is that everyone experiences pain, the pain of isolation, the pain of separation, the pain of loneliness or whatever form it comes in. And, I am becoming increasingly convinced that a sense of isolation is at the root of many self-destructive behaviors and of the chronic emotional stress that can lead to diseases like heart disease."

□ 14 □

2020: A Heart Disease Odyssey

Just as you and I have benefited—and doesn't that word seem weak here?—from the information, techniques and procedures we have been discussing, so will the next generation have the advantage of the research and development that is taking place now. It is important to remember that most of our knowledge of the diagnosis and treatment of heart disease has been developed in the past thirty years or so. Just think what the next comparable period should bring!

The gene for atherosclerosis has been located on chromosome 19p, although its exact location has so far defied searchers. That gene is associated with low levels of HDL cholesterol; high levels of triglycerides; and high levels of small, dense particles of LDL cholesterol, a pattern called ATHS. As many as one person in three is thought to have this defect, and when a test is developed to identify them before onset of the disease, much will be prevented by diet, drug, or exercise therapy.

Two diagnostic tools show enormous promise: the first is a variation on the CT (or "Cat") scan and is called Ultrafast CT (CT stands for computed tomography). The heart beats too fast to provide anything but a blurred image in a conventional Cat scan, but by speeding up the

scanning by a factor of from 10 to 20, clear "pictures"—
they are actually computer-generated images—can be
obtained. The advantage of this technology could be
beyond measure: since it is noninvasive its use is free of
risk, so many asymptomatic people could be examined.
One must not forget that for many of the more than 1.5
million people who have heart attacks in the United States
each year, the first symptom is death.

The second method is called intravascular ultrasound.
This tool involves a catheter, much like angiography, and
produces very clear images of the interior of the arteries
where it is guided. This method allows for the identification of soft plaques or other arterial damage that might
elude other techniques.

Once the effects of disease have been located, there
will be several new methods of dealing with them. Much
of coronary artery bypass graft surgery may be replaced
by laser surgery, whereby a catheter will be used to
introduce a laser beam to "zap" the offending atheromas
and leave the vessel walls undamaged. The technique for
this is ready and only awaits the discovery or development
of a gas whose burning will destroy *only* the plaque and
its accumulated debris. An advantage of this method, in
addition to the obvious ones of comfort and cost, is that
the material of the plaque would be vaporized.

Another use of the laser is in experimental use already.
Acting on the principle that the freshest blood is within the
heart itself (on the left side, where it comes into the atrium
after oxygenation in the lungs, flows into the ventricle, and
is ejected to the body), trans-myocardial revascularization
uses large numbers of minute laser beam pulses to make
tiny channels *within* the heart. The entrance and exit holes
are sufficiently small to seal themselves. The model is of the
heart as rubber foam sponge, say, not as inflated balloon.

The hypothesis is that fresh blood should then be able to circulate freely, in quantities sufficient to benefit the heart's tissues but not so great as to cause harm by inappropriate accumulation. Early reports are enthusiastic, as early reports frequently are.

As we saw earlier, the chief liability of angioplasty is that restenosis, or collapse of the artery, occurs about 40 percent of the time, thereby requiring a repetition of the procedure or bypass surgery; sometimes the collapse can cause a heart attack. The placing of a small supporting metal coil, or stent, in the artery at the place of angioplasty has been shown to reduce the rate of restenosis by about one-third.

Most muscle tissue is capable of regeneration, but heart tissue is not. The tissue affected by a heart attack quickly dies of starvation. In experiments with laboratory mice, fetal heart muscle tissue was transplanted into adult heart muscle that had undergone infarction and, dramatically, it was shown to promote regeneration of tissue. We are probably a long way from similar experiments with human beings, but the suggestions and possibilities raised on both a practical and a theoretical level are very provocative indeed.

Here's one you should like: the descendants of a couple who lived in Limone, Italy, in the eighteenth century have a simple mutation in a protein that is part of their HDL cholesterol and which protects them from the fatty deposits that might otherwise clog their arteries. This mutation is called Apoliprotein A-1 Milano and it is conceivable that it could be introduced into the bodies of particularly vulnerable people where it would reproduce itself and offer similar immunity.

And here is my favorite, although I can offer few details. A machine somewhat like a giant blood pressure cuff and looking like the bottom half of a space suit inflates and deflates in a rhythm opposite to that of the heart, inflating while the heart is at rest between beats. This pushes the blood into the heart and thereby promotes the growth of new blood vessels around the damaging blockages, a process called collateralization. This technique is called enhanced external counterpulsation and, while invented in the United States, it was perfected and used extensively in China. It has been shown to be highly effective in reducing angina without drugs or surgery. While only experimental in the United States at the present time, it is to be hoped that it will become widely available soon.

Most important of all, however, will be the three saving factors: prevention, prevention, prevention. Our knowledge of heart or coronary artery disease increases every day, and evidence against significant risk factors accumulates. People with a hereditary predisposition to the disease will be tested earlier and more easily and appropriate precautions taken; despite the tobacco industry's desperate efforts to the contrary, cigarette smoking will be all but eliminated from much of the world, thereby also eliminating the active and passive damage it causes; healthy exercise will be more widely taken, a trend already well underway (thirty years ago, did you ever see a sixty-year-old jogging?); diet will be dramatically improved by developments in the preservation and transportation of food. We don't know yet what causes cancer or a number of other scourges of mankind, but the origins of heart disease, the single biggest cause of death in this country, are known, identifiable, and can be avoided. It would be nice to think that fifty years from now a medical historian will look back on our time and think of heart disease as a quaint, exotic—and eradicated—plague.

□ 15 □

Farewell

In the event you have not come to this conclusion on your own, I will spell it out for you: you have been—or soon will be—given a new life. I said early on how lucky you are to be having these problems now, and maybe that's getting through. Thirty years ago there was no bypass surgery; twenty-five years ago there was very little ITA graft surgery; fifteen years ago we did not know the benefits of aspirin; ten years ago there was no Mevacor. In my memory, heart disease was treated with prolonged bed rest; today it is treated with exercise. Not so long ago it virtually ended your life; now it begins it. We learn more now about the causes of heart disease and its treatment every day. Think what it will be like in thirty more years!

It is tempting to think of ourselves as "cured," but vigilance is the key for a long and healthy future. To prevent recurrence (or indeed initial problems), here is an outline of what we have learned. It is the secret to heart health. Follow it—please.

1. *Quit smoking cigarettes.*
2. *Establish a diet that is satisfying to you and stick to it.*
3. *Establish the ideal range of your weight and stay within it.*

4. *Keep your total cholesterol below 200.*

5. *Keep the ratio of your total cholesterol to HDL cholesterol below 5.*

6. *Limit your consumption of alcohol to two drinks per day.*

7. *Exercise regularly, with a goal of expending two thousand calories per week, most of it dynamic or cardiovascular.*

8. *Follow the course of medication prescribed by your doctor.*

9. *To the greatest degree possible, identify the sources of emotional stress in your life and avoid them,*

10. *And the corollary, seek the worthwhile activities that give you real joy and satisfaction and pursue them.*

11. *Use your new life as a gift—which it is.*

A lot of people went to a lot of effort to get you here. Take care.

APPENDIX

A Brief History of Coronary Artery Bypass Surgery

In our culture we tend to romanticize the creative process and are inclined to think of momentous discoveries or inventions as the work of a single person, much like a great work of art. In science, medicine, or surgery this is very seldom true. Innovations in these fields develop over time and work on the principle of O.T.S.O.G., On The Shoulders Of Giants: it is easier to see over a high fence when you are standing on the shoulders of giants.

This is not to minimize the accomplishments of any one person but to point out that the source of important innovations is not a vacuum but a history of inspiration, imagination, effort, experiment, error, failure—and persistence, even in the face of doubt and skepticism. The history of coronary artery bypass surgery is a relatively brief one but is important for you to know because each of its major contributors gave you a present more generous and needed than anything else in your life: your second chance. It was suggested earlier that we tip our hats to them; now let's raise a great cheer!

The chronological baseline is as recent as 1863, when Theodor Billroth (1829–1894), the Viennese pioneer abdominal surgeon recognized as initiating the modern era of surgery, wrote, "Any surgeon who wishes to preserve the respect of his colleagues would never attempt to suture the heart." Tissue must not be moving when it is sutured, especially tissue as delicate and vulnerable as the heart's; a still heart means death; therefore the heart is out of bounds. Period.

This was the attitude that prevailed of necessity during the early decades of this century, even as more was being learned about coronary heart disease and the invalids it produced. But how could the living heart be studied? In 1929, a young German physician, Werner Forssmann (1904–1979), believed he could thread a catheter into a heart so that dye (for an X ray) could be injected or measurements taken. His superiors in the clinic in Eberswald, Germany, where he worked, forbade his attempts at so dangerous an experiment. Needing both an assistant and access to sterile instruments, he enlisted a nurse as an accomplice and persuaded her to be the experimental subject. He gained entry to the operating room at an off-hour, strapped his "subject" securely to the surgical table, and then proceeded to open a vein, insert the catheter, and guide it into the heart—*of himself!* He then released the nurse so that she could accompany him to the radiology laboratory and help him take the X ray that would prove what he had accomplished.

His success at this first catheterization was confirmed, and the doors to the future of cardiology were opened. No longer was the heart forbidden territory. Forssmann was to receive the Nobel Prize in Medicine twenty-seven years later, aware of his accomplishment but wondering what all the fuss was about. Instead of a high-profile medical career, he chose to spend his life caring for the people of a small town.

By the mid 1930s the American surgeon Claude S. Beck (1894–1971) had identified a solution to the symptoms of heart disease as revascularization, a new source of blood. He had read the report of a post-mortem examination of a man who had had extensive heart disease but who had thrived because his heart, or myocardium, had adhered to his pericardium, its protective sac, and developed a completely new source of blood. Beck tried to induce similar adhesions in the operating room with a number of different methods: irritation of the surface of the heart and pericardium by abrasion with rough surfaces or by putting powdered talc in the pericardium (called poudrage), and making pedicles of muscle, omentum, spleen, stomach, and the like. It sounds grotesque to us today, but here is an example of his results: In one study of thirty-seven patients after six years, fourteen had died soon after surgery (whether from the surgery or the preexisting condition is not known), nine had died during the six years (again, it is not recorded from what), but fourteen had done very well and were thriving. Certainly the procedure was not without risk, but what other hope did they have? Dr. Beck spent his whole medical career at Case Western Reserve University in Cleveland, Ohio.

In 1945, the Canadian surgeon Arthur M. Vineberg (1903–1988) at McGill University in Montreal published the suggestion that the nearby internal mammary artery, now known as the internal thoracic artery or ITA, be used as the new source of blood, and in a number of surgical procedures he implanted the freely bleeding end of the artery into the left ventricular myocardium, hoping the heart would take advantage of this new blood source. Often it did, and reasonable success was achieved. Indeed, a recent (1991) report told of patients in their seventies and eighties with such implants doing well after more than twenty-five years.

Like a bar on the door, though, further progress was impeded by the inability to stop the heart during surgery;

a number of efforts were made to develop a successful heart-lung machine, and finally on May 6, 1953, John H. Gibbon, Jr., at Jefferson Medical College in Philadelphia, was rewarded for his many years of devotion to this research. On that day, he performed the first successful surgery on a human patient using cardiopulmonary bypass. Stopping the heart altogether, he was able to repair a large hole between the right and left atria, called an atrial septal defect, of an eighteen-year-old girl. Also during this decade, Mason Sones (1919–1985) at the Cleveland Clinic in Ohio, was devoting his extraordinary energy and skills to the extension of Forssmann's pioneer use of the cardiac catheter. Dr. Sones's goal was to make clear and useful *selective* images, both moving and still, of the heart and its arteries, and this he succeeded in doing for the first time on October 24, 1958. With these two new technologies it was only a matter of time before both surgical techniques and sufficient knowledge—and control—of the body's chemistry were developed. Coronary bypass surgery as a choice for the relief of the symptoms of coronary heart disease was on the horizon.

And the first time such surgery was performed was unplanned. On August 31, 1964, a forty-two-year-old man was admitted to the Methodist Hospital in Houston, Texas, with severe angina pectoris—indeed, so severe that he had been unable to work for almost a year. Subsequent tests and arteriograms showed extensive disease. It was believed, however, that nothing could be done beyond medication and rest, so the patient was discharged with instructions to take his medicine and restrict his activity. His condition deteriorated and he was readmitted to the hospital on November 16, unable to even walk without pain. In the absence of Michael DeBakey, the chief of surgery, H. Edward Garrett, later of the University of

Tennessee, decided to perform an operation called a coronary endarterectomy, in which fatty deposits and other occlusions are surgically removed from the coronary arteries. The operation was scheduled for November 23.

All went according to plan until the patient's coronary arteries were inspected; it turned out that disease was so severe and diffuse that endarterectomy would be far too much of a risk for the little that might be gained. Because the patient had no hope of regaining a tolerable life without some drastic improvement in his heart's blood supply, Dr. Garrett decided to try something never attempted before: Using a length of reversed saphenous vein from the patient's leg, he would create a bypass from the aorta to the left anterior descending coronary artery, above the highest blockage. It worked. In Dr. Garrett's own words, "The operation was accomplished without incident, and convalescence after operation was uncomplicated." The patient was able to return to work and was thriving seven years later when an extensive series of follow-up studies was carried out.

This should have been one of those very rare events, a single incident that changed the course of history. It is to be regretted that this was not the case. When Dr. DeBakey returned to Houston and saw the astounding results of the procedure, he directed that three patients with a similar disease be found for surgery. He performed surgical bypasses on each of them, and each of them died. He directed that no further attempts at coronary artery bypass surgery be made in Methodist Hospital and spoke out against such surgery. Indeed, the successful—and *extraordinary* is not too strong a word—discovery by Dr. Garrett was not even reported until 1973, when an article appeared in the *Journal of the American Medical Association*. This was *more than eight years* after the event. One can only speculate about what might have taken place in coronary bypass surgery had it been published in a timely fashion.

Fully reported and well documented, though, was a similar procedure carried out at the Cleveland Clinic on May 9, 1967 by the Argentine surgeon René G. Favoloro. He is quite widely, albeit inaccurately, credited with performing this surgery for the first time, but neither he nor anyone else at the time knew otherwise. He and the team at the Cleveland Clinic pioneered and developed the technique and deserve full credit for it. (Columbus was not the first European to visit the New World, either.)

Inspired by Vineberg's work and convinced that an independent blood supply was critical to long-term patency, George E. Green, then at New York University, performed a number of successful coronary artery bypasses on laboratory dogs using the internal thoracic artery, and in February of 1968 performed a coronary artery bypass on a human patient with the ITA for the first time, at the New York Veteran's Administration Hospital. That procedure, somewhat more demanding on the surgeon than the saphenous vein bypass, has proved itself over the years to be the bypass operation of choice. To quote from the *Year Book of Cardiology* for 1989 in a review of an article on the subject, "Internal mammary artery bypass grafting was an independent predictor of survival; use of this graft reduced the risk of dying by a factor of 0.64. The internal mammary artery bypass graft is the vessel of choice for coronary artery disease. Its use should be considered for any subgroup of patients."

Heaven only knows how many millions of arterial or venous bypasses have been done since 1967. We "veterans," whether when we are on our way to the gym or getting ready to run a marathon or just playing with our grandchildren, have these great physicians to thank for it.

Glossary

ACE inhibitors Short for angiotensin-converting enzyme inhibitors, a class of drugs that improves vascular blood flow by inhibiting the production of the hormone angiotensin II, which constricts the blood vessels. Examples are Capoten, Prinivil, and Vasotec.

Acids, trans fatty Artificially produced dietary substances formed during conversion of vegetable oils to shortenings or margarine which are solid at room temperature; they act like, and are as harmful as, saturated fats, and raise levels of LDL cholesterol.

Alpha-blockers Short for alpha-adrenergic blocking drugs; a class of drugs used to control HYPERTENSION by acting on the ALPHA RECEPTORS that control dilation of the vessels. Examples are Cardura, Hytrin, and Minipress.

Alpha receptors A group of cells in blood vessels that control dilation.

Anastomosis In surgery, the artificial joining of two tubular organs; in heart surgery, the grafting of a VEIN or ARTERY to a coronary artery or aorta.

Anemia A condition of reduced quantities of HEMO-GLOBIN in the red blood cells, resulting in increased fatigue and diminished resistance to infection.

Anesthesiologist A physician who designs and executes the program of anesthesia during surgery and also monitors body function and response during that time.

Angina pectoris Literally, strangulation of the chest. A condition which is caused by narrowing of the CORONARY ARTERIES that supply blood to the heart, resulting in a temporary "starvation" of the heart for blood. Symptoms are sudden pains in the chest and/or upper body; a constricted or congested feeling in the area of the heart; and pronounced feelings of doom. Characteristic of the most common form, stable angina, is the "controllability" of the symptoms: disappearance with brief rest and reappearance with a specific amount of exercise. Unstable angina is less predictable, is usually considered more serious, and is also known as preinfarction (preheart attack) angina; and PRINZMETAL ANGINA is unpredictable, occurring even at rest, and is caused by CORONARY SPASM. When the spasm is relieved, little or no residual blockage or obstruction remains in the coronary artery. Angina pectoris is the principal indication of the presence of coronary artery or heart disease.

Angiogram An image of an ARTERY made by ANGIO-GRAPHY.

Angiography The procedure by which a thin, flexible tube or CATHETER is introduced into an ARTERY in the arm or groin and guided toward and into the CORONARY ARTERIES and the heart itself. Opaque dye is injected and recording devices produce an image on a fluoroscope screen, still, movie film, or videotape.

Angioplasty A procedure in which a thin, flexible tube or CATHETER is introduced into an ARTERY in the arm or groin and guided into a CORONARY ARTERY. In balloon angioplasty, this is done with a specially designed catheter with an inflatable section near the tip; when in position above an obstruction in the coronary artery, it is inflated and the obstruction depressed, thus widening the artery.

Anticoagulant A drug that delays coagulation, or "clotting," of the blood.

Antihypertensive agent   A drug used to lower the blood pressure; general categories are tranquilizers, blood vessel relaxants, and diuretics.

Antioxidants   Substances that inhibit the oxidation of LDL cholesterol, perhaps thereby slowing the development of heart disease; vitamins C and E, carotene, and riboflavin are the principal ones.

Aorta   The large artery which is the initial conduit of freshly oxygenated blood from the heart to the rest of the body.

Aortic valve   The three-lobed valve between the left ventricle of the heart and the aorta, through which passes the recently oxygenated blood from the heart to the rest of the body by way of the arteries.

Aortocoronary bypass   Bypass made from the aorta to a coronary artery, most commonly made with a section of vein, usually the SAPHENOUS VEIN, but occasionally with a length of artery; an example of a FREE GRAFT.

Apoliprotein A-1 Milano   Genetic mutation in HDL cholesterol which protects arteries from ATHEROSCLEROSIS; it is found among descendants of a couple who lived in Limone, Italy, in the eighteenth century.

Apoprotein   Molecule carried by the LIPOPROTEIN that eases the chemical process of mixing the lipoprotein with the blood.

Arrhythmia   Irregularity in the otherwise predictable rhythm of the heartbeat.

Arteriogram   See ANGIOGRAM.

Arteriography   See ANGIOGRAPHY.

Arteriole   The very small branch of an ARTERY that supplies blood to the CAPILLARIES.

Arteriosclerosis   Hardening of any of the arteries by disease.

Artery   A blood vessel that takes oxygenated blood *away from* the heart to the rest of the body.

Atheroma   A mass, usually of fatty substances, that builds up on the wall of an artery, intrudes into, and scars the artery itself and impedes the flow of blood through the artery.

Atherosclerosis   A form of ARTERIOSCLEROSIS affecting the arteries carrying blood to the heart, brain, kidneys, legs, and arms.

ATHS   A pattern of low levels of HDL cholesterol, high levels of TRIGLYCERIDES, and high levels of small, dense particles of LDL cholesterol.

Atrioventricular bundle   The conduit for a signal to contract from the ATRIOVENTRICULAR NODE to the VENTRICLES.

Atrioventricular node   A mass of modified heart muscle in the lower middle part of the right ATRIUM that controls the contraction of the atrium and sends a signal to the VENTRICLES to contract by way of the ATRIOVENTRICULAR BUNDLE.

Atrium   One of the two upper chambers of the heart; the *right* atrium receives deoxygenated blood from the body by way of the VENAE CAVAE and pumps it into the right VENTRICLE; the *left* atrium receives oxygenated blood from the lungs through the PULMONARY vein and pumps it into the left ventricle.

Auricle   A small pouch in the wall of each atrium of the heart. The word is sometimes used synonomously but incorrectly for the ATRIUM.

AV node   See ATRIOVENTRICULAR NODE.

Balloon angioplasty   See ANGIOPLASTY.

Beta-blockers   Beta-adrenergic blocking drugs, a group of drugs that prevent stimulation of certain receptors of the sympathetic nervous system, used to control HYPER-TENSION. They also slow and regulate the beating of the heart, reduce its need for oxygen, and thereby reduce ANGINA. Examples are Kerlone, Lopressor, Tenormin, and Inderal.

Beta receptors Beta-adrenergic receptors of the sympathetic nervous system which are stimulated by hormones produced during exercise or emotional stress.

Bilateral grafts See GRAFTS, BILATERAL.

Brachial artery An artery extending from the armpit to the inner side of the elbow.

Bradycardia An abnormally slow heartbeat.

CABG Pronounced "cabbage." An abbreviation for CORONARY ARTERY BYPASS GRAFT surgery, a procedure in which either the lower end of the INTERNAL THORACIC ARTERY is dissected away from the chest wall and grafted to the coronary artery below the blockage, thus providing a supply of blood from a new source; or a section of SAPHENOUS VEIN is removed from the leg and grafted around the blockage. Frequently a combination of these two procedures is used.

Calcium channel-blockers or **calcium antagonists** A group of drugs that impede constriction of the CORONARY ARTERIES and also widen the arteries in the rest of the body, thereby allowing a greater and more efficient flow of blood. They are also used to treat high blood pressure, HYPERTENSION. Examples are Calan, Cardizem, Norvasc, Procardia, and Verelan.

Capillary The tiny blood vessels that are the farthest extent of the vascular system; they are supplied with blood by the end of the system of arteries, ARTERIOLES, and drained by VENULES, the smallest part of the system of veins.

Cardiac   Of or pertaining to the heart.

Cardiac arrest   Stopping of the heartbeat, usually because of interference with the electrical impulses that regulate it.

Cardiac ultrasound   See ECHOCARDIOGRAM.

Cardiology   The medical study of the heart, both healthy and diseased.

Cardioplegia solution   A solution of chemicals used to stop the heart during surgery.

Cardiopulmonary bypass machine   The technical name for the HEART-LUNG MACHINE.

Cardiovascular or **circulatory**   Pertaining to the system that delivers oxygen- and nutrition-enriched blood to the body's tissues, returns oxygen-poor blood to the heart and lungs, and removes waste products for ultimate disposal.

Cardioversion   The use of electricity to restore normal rhythm to the heart.

Catheter   A small, hollow, flexible tube that is used to either introduce or drain fluids. In cardiac CATHETERIZATION the tube is guided into the coronary arteries from either the arm or the groin and dye and radio-opaque dye is released, thus allowing images of the coronary arteries to be recorded.

Catheterization   The examination of the heart with a CATHETER.

Cholesterol   One of the two major types of fat in the blood, the other being TRIGLYCERIDES; technically a steroid, it is found in all animal fats and manufactured in the liver. It is one of the essential building elements of the human body but is also potentially harmful when present in excess. It does not dissolve in blood and is carried to the tissues as part of a complex molecule called a LIPOPROTEIN; it may leave the molecule and build up on the wall of an artery, forming a PLAQUE or ATHEROMA. Measured in milligrams of cholesterol per 100 milliliters of blood plasma (liquid), normal levels are 150 to 180 and (decreasingly) acceptable levels extend up to 230.

Chylomicron A complex fat molecule that carries CHOLESTEROL in the blood.

Cineangiography The technique of filming opaque dye in its passage through blood vessels.

Circulatory system The whole system whose function is to circulate blood: the VEINS, ARTERIES, and heart.

Coagulation The clotting of the blood.

Collateral circulation The development of tiny arteries around an arterial blockage as an alternative blood supply to a section of the heart.

Collateralization The development of secondary blood vessels as the primary ones become blocked.

Coronary artery Any of the four principal blood vessels that supply oxygen-rich blood to the heart muscle itself, primarily the left ventricle. They are: (1) the left main (LMCA), with its two branches; (2) left anterior descending (LAD); (3) left circumflex (LCA); and (4) the right coronary artery (RCA). From the right coronary artery branches a minor artery, the posterior descending artery.

Coronary artery bypass graft (CABG) The use of blood vessels to provide a fresh supply of blood to the heart, or REVASCULARIZE.

Coronary artery disease A disease of the CORONARY ARTERIES, where CHOLESTEROL and other LIPIDS accumulate to form a PLAQUE or ATHEROMA and impede the flow of blood to the heart muscle or MYOCARDIUM.

Coronary flow reserve The measurement of blood flow to the heart.

Coronary heart disease The symptoms and features of CORONARY ARTERY DISEASE.

Coronary occlusion An obstruction of one of the CORONARY ARTERIES that slows or stops blood supply to the heart tissue.

Coronary spasm A sudden contraction in a segment of the CORONARY ARTERY, obstructing flow of blood to the heart muscle, the same as if by blockage. There is increased danger of INFARCTION if the artery is already blocked, a narrowing of an already narrow conduit. Mysterious as to source, it is associated with emotional stress.

Coronary thrombosis CORONARY OCCLUSION caused by a blood clot.

Counterpulsation, enhanced external A technique carried out with a mechanism similar to a large blood pressure cuff and put over the lower half of the body; it constricts in a rhythm opposite to that of the heart, forcing blood back to the heart and thereby encouraging COLLATERALIZATION.

CT, Ultrafast Computed tomography ("Cat scan") done at a speed sufficient to produce clear and usable images of a beating heart.

Diastole The period when the VENTRICLES relax and refill with blood. The pressure at this time is called DIASTOLIC and is measured in millimeters of mercury; it is the second or lower of the two numbers that measure the blood pressure, the first being the SYSTOLIC.

Diastolic pressure See DIASTOLE.

Diuretic A drug that promotes urine excretion.

Dynamic exercise Continuing exercise over a period of time that calls on the heart to do more work to deliver oxygen to the tissues. The purpose is to increase the rate or number of heartbeats per minute and to sustain the higher level for a reasonable period of time. In time, the heart will deliver the same amount of oxygen at a lower level and therefore will be more efficient. Also called cardiovasclur, C.V., and aerobic exercise, it is to be contrasted to STATIC EXERCISE.

Echocardiogram A noninvasive test in which high-frequency sound waves are used to measure size and thickness of various parts of the heart. The information produced is in the form of a picture on a monitor or a graph on paper. Also called CARDIAC ULTRASOUND.

Eicosapentaenoic acid An OMEGA-3 FATTY ACID.

Ejection fraction Measured in percent (of the capacity of the left ventricle), the amount of blood pushed out of the heart with each heartbeat, a measure of the heart's efficiency.

EKG Abbreviation for ELECTROCARDIOGRAM.

Electrocardiogram The graph on paper that is the result of electrocardiography, the recording of the electrical activity of the heart at rest. It is an extremely important tool in the diagnosis of heart disease.

Endarterectomy The surgical removal of arterial plaque deposits.

Endocarditis An infection, usually bacterial, of one or more of the heart valves, the ENDOCARDIUM; it requires intensive antibiotic therapy and frequently ends up requiring heart valve replacement.

Endocardium The delicate membrane that lines the heart.

Endotracheal tube A tube placed into the trachea or windpipe through the mouth, used to facilitate control and content of air breathed, particularly during surgery.

EPA EICOSAPENTAENOIC ACID, an OMEGA-3 FATTY ACID.

Epicardium   The outermost layer of the heart wall.

Exercise   Activity or physical exertion whose goal is body conditioning, fitness, or correction; aerobic, cardiovascular, and DYNAMIC all refer to continuous exercise whose purpose is to elevate heart rate and maintain that rate at a higher level in order to increase cardiac efficiency; STATIC EXERCISE is sporadic and may put stress on a vulnerable heart.

Exercise EKG   An ELECTROCARDIOGRAM done during exercise, usually on a treadmill; it provides information about blood flow to the heart muscle during activity. This is also called a stress test.

Fats (saturation)   A molecule of fat is said to be saturated or unsaturated depending on the number of hydrogen atoms attached to it; the more hydrogen atoms, the more saturated it is. Unsaturated fats are divided into monounsaturated and polyunsaturated depending on the number of places on the molecule available to hydrogen atoms. Characteristics and sources of these fats are:
Saturated: Solid at room temperature; stimulates the manufacture of LDL ("bad") cholesterol. Sources: animal fats, eggs, offal, coconut oil, chocolate.
Monounsaturated: Liquid at room temperature; lowers cholesterol levels without reducing HDL ("good") cholesterol. Sources: olive oil, canola oil, avocados.
Polyunsaturated: Liquid at room temperature; lowers levels of HDL cholesterol *and* LDL cholesterol; high in calories. Sources: vegetable oils and margarine.

Femoral artery   An artery starting at the hip and running two-thirds of the way down the front of the thigh and then passing into the back of the thigh and behind the knee.

Fibrillation   Abnormally fast and irregular heartbeat;

atrial fibrillation, that of the heart's upper chambers, is not uncommon in cases of heart disease and is evidenced by a very rapid and irregular pulse and heartbeat. The heart can be restored to normal rhythm either by the administration of digoxin or by electric shock, CARDIOVERSION. Ventricular fibrillation, which occurs in the lower chambers, is usually produced by a heart attack and causes the heart to stop beating, resulting in death. This is called Sudden Death Syndrome.

Fluoroscope An instrument by which X-ray images may be viewed directly, rather than with the more common use of film.

Fluvastatin One of the STATINS, and sold under the brand name LESCOL.

Foley catheter A tube placed in the urinary bladder to collect urine and prevent incontinence.

Framingham study An epidemiological study of heart disease and its causes, initially carried out among 5,127 members of the population of Framingham, Massachusetts. The original study group was every other male and female between the ages of thirty and sixty who exhibited no symptoms of heart disease. It was begun in 1948 by a team from Boston University Medical School and continues to this day among the offspring of the original group.

Free radicals Highly reactive fatty compounds which are the likely cause of PLAQUE development and growth.

French Paradox Why do the French, with a diet high in fat, have a 40 percent lower rate of coronary heart disease than the Americans? See RESVERATROL.

Graft
    arterial The use of an ARTERY to provide a new source of blood to the heart.

free The use of a segment of artery or VEIN to make a bypass, usually from the AORTA to the CORONARY ARTERY between the obstruction and the heart.

pedicled The use of one end of an artery, usually the INTERNAL THORACIC or ITA to provide a new supply of blood to the heart; the other end remains intact, thus providing blood from a fresh source.

vein The use of a segment of vein to make a free graft.

Grafts

bilateral The use of the INTERNAL THORACIC ARTERY on each side for grafts.

sequential The use of a single length of VEIN or ARTERY to make two or more grafts.

HDL High Density Lipoprotein, a molecule that picks up cholesterol in the tissues and carries it to the liver for eventual excretion. The "good" molecule, it helps to protect against the development of ATHEROSCLEROSIS. An important source is fresh saltwater fish.

Hmg-CoA reductase inhibitors See STATINS.

Heart attack Death of heart tissue due to lack of blood supply; MYOCARDIAL INFARCTION.

Heart-lung machine A machine that carries out the functions of oxygenating and pumping the blood, normally performed by the heart and lungs, while the heart is being repaired.

Hematocrit The volume of red blood cells (erythrocytes) in the blood, expressed as a percentage. The number is obtained by centrifuging the blood sample in a tube and measuring the packed cells against the total.

Hemoglobin The blood protein that carries oxygen to the body's tissues.

Heparin An anticoagulant or "blood thinner" used to prevent clotting during heart surgery.

Heredity   The transmission of characteristics from parent to offspring through the genes.

High blood pressure   See HYPERTENSION.

High Density Lipoprotein   See HDL.

Holter monitor   A portable and wearable EKG machine that records the electrical activity of the heart over an extended period of time.

Hypertension   Elevated blood pressure, which increases both the work of the heart and the risk of developing heart disease.

Infarct   An area of tissue, especially in the heart, that has died for lack of blood. MYOCARDIAL INFARCTION is the technical term for "heart attack."

Internal mammary artery   A commonly used term for the INTERNAL THORACIC ARTERY.

Internal thoracic artery (ITA)   Known as the internal mammary artery until its renaming in 1955 and still frequently referred to as such, the two internal thoracic arteries arise from the subclavian arteries just above the first rib and descend inside the chest cavity to the sixth rib. The location and resistance to ATHEROSCLEROSIS of these arteries make them appropriate for CORONARY ARTERY BYPASS GRAFT surgery.

Intravascular ultrasound   An invasive method of imaging, using sound to produce clear pictures of the interior of arteries.

Intravenous (I.V.)   Placed into a vein, as an injection or a catheter.

Ischemia   A condition where tissue suffers from an inadequate supply of blood, caused by blockage or constriction of the blood vessel supplying it.

Ischemic heart disease   See CORONARY HEART DISEASE.

Jugular vein   One of three large veins in the neck that drain blood from the brain, scalp, face, and neck.

LDL   Low Density Lipoprotein, a molecule that transports cholesterol and tends to deposit it on arterial walls. The "bad" molecule associated with the buildup of PLAQUES or ATHEROMAS, whose chief source is animal fats. Animal organ meats, such as sweetbreads and liver, are particularly rich in LDL molecules.

Lescol   The brand name of FLUVASTATIN; see STATINS.

Lifestyle Heart Trial   A year-long trial devised and supervised by Dr. Dean Ornish in which the results of drastic heart disease risk-factor reduction (particularly diet, stress reduction, and exercise) were compared to the results of moderate reduction.

Lipid   A fat that is not soluble in the blood.

Lipoprotein   A complex molecule of a specific type found in blood plasma that attaches itself to and transports fats and other lipid molecules. See HDL, LDL, and VLDL.

Lovastatin   One of the STATINS, and sold under the brand name MEVACOR.

Low Density Lipoprotein   See LDL.

Lumen   The space enclosed by a tubular or saclike organ; in this context, the interior of a blood vessel through which blood flows and which may become constricted by disease.

Lung   One of the pair of organs in the chest cavity behind the heart whose function is to cleanse the blood of waste gases, which it expels in respiration, and to oxygenate it for return to the body by way of the heart.

Mammary artery   The former name for the INTERNAL THORACIC ARTERY.

Median sternotomy   See STERNOTOMY, MEDIAN.

Mended Hearts   An association of heart surgery patients whose purpose is to provide support and disseminate information.

Mevacor The brand name of LOVASTATIN; see STATINS.

Mitral valve In the heart, the VALVE between the left ATRIUM and the left VENTRICLE; also called the bicuspid valve, because of its two flaps.

Monounsaturated fats See FATS (SATURATION).

Myocardial infarction The death of heart muscle tissue due to a cessation of blood supply.

Myocardium The middle of the three layers that form the wall of the heart; the muscular layer.

Nasogastric tube A tube placed into the stomach through the nose.

Nitrate A salt or ester of nitric acid; specifically, a chemical agent used to dilate blood vessels.

Nitroglycerin A drug that dilates or expands the blood vessels and is frequently used to alleviate the discomfort of ANGINA PECTORIS.

Obesity The condition of being significantly overweight, usually 20 percent or more above ideal body weight.

Occlusion The obstruction or closing of a blood vessel.

Omega-3 fatty acids EICOSAPENTAENOIC and docosahexaenoic acids, found in fish oils. They lower blood levels of TRIGLYCERIDES; they reduce the stickiness of blood PLATELETS, the cells that initiate clotting, and inhibit the formation of fibrinogen, which is an important protein in COAGULATION, thereby reducing heart attack and stroke; and they may help to prevent ventricular FIBRILLATION.

Open heart surgery Surgery performed on or in the heart with the help of the HEART-LUNG MACHINE.

Oxidation Chemical process in which oxygen atoms become attached to unstable molecules. It is believed that the oxidation of LDL cholesterol makes it more easily deposited on arterial walls and that this process is hindered by ANTIOXIDANTS.

Oxygen free-radicals Highly reactive, unstable molecules that act on LDL cholesterol by OXIDATION and begin the process of PLAQUE formation.

Pacemaker Electrical device that maintains a normal heartbeat for the patient by stimulating the surface of the ventricle. The device itself can be outside of the body or be surgically implanted under a person's skin.

Palpitation Fluttering feeling in the heart.

Patency The quality of being PATENT; one might speak of the degree of patency.

Patent Open or unobstructed, as in a grafted artery or vein.

Pedicle graft See GRAFT, pedicle.

Percutaneous Through the skin.

Percutaneous Transluminal Coronary Angioplasty See ANGIOPLASTY.

Perfusion The passage of blood through lung tissue for oxidation, hence the oxidation of blood in the CARDIOPULMONARY BYPASS, or HEART-LUNG MACHINE.

Perfusionist The technician who operates the HEART-LUNG MACHINE.

Pericarditis An inflammation of the PERICARDIUM.

Pericardium The membranous sac that surrounds and protects the heart.

Plaque A fatty deposit in a blood vessel, also called an ATHEROMA.

Platelets An important component of the blood. Disc-shaped, their several functions all relate to COAGULATION.

Polyunsaturated fats   See FATS (SATURATION)

Pravachol   The brand name of PRAVASTATIN; see STATINS.

Pravastatin   One of the STATINS, and sold under the brand name PRAVACHOL.

Prinzmetal angina   In contrast to stable angina, Prinzmetal is unpredictable and not induced by exertion. Named for Myron Prinzmetal, who first described it, it frequently occurs at night or in the early morning when the sufferer is at rest; its pain and other discomfort is every bit as vivid as that from stable angina.

PTCA   PERCUTANEOUS TRANSLUMINAL CORONARY ANGIOPLASTY; see ANGIOPLASTY.

Pulmonary   Of or relating to the lungs.

Pulmonary artery   The artery that takes blood from the heart to the lungs for oxygenation.

Pulmonic valve   The valve in the heart between the right VENTRICLE and the PULMONARY ARTERY.

Radial artery   A branch of the BRACHIAL ARTERY that runs from the elbow to the inside of the wrist.

Reactive oxygen species   Unstable molecules produced by the body that stabilize themselves by attachment to fat molecules, among other substances, a process called OXIDATION; this process can alter the structure and function of the target molecule drastically.

Restenosis   The repeated narrowing of a previously expanded artery.

Resveratrol   A substance found in all grapes but particularly the Concord, it reduces levels of cholesterol and the clumping of blood cells that leads to ATHEROSCLEROSIS and heart attack; it may be the source of the FRENCH PARADOX.

Revascularization   The provision of a new supply of

blood, as with an ARTERIAL or VEIN GRAFT to the CORO-
NARY ARTERY.

SA node   SINOATRIAL NODE.

Saphenous vein   The longest vein in the body, extending
from the foot up the inside of the leg to the groin;
sections of this vein are often used for CORONARY
BYPASSES.

Saturated fats   See FATS (SATURATION).

Sequential grafts   See GRAFTS, SEQUENTIAL.

Sestamibi Stress Test   An EXERCISE EKG similar to the
THALLIUM STRESS TEST but using the radioactive tracer
Sestamibi.

Simvastatin   One of the STATINS, and sold under the
brand name ZOCOR.

Sinoatrial node   A microscopic area of specialized heart
muscle in the upper wall of the right ATRIUM that sends
electrical signals to control the heartbeat.

Spasm, coronary   See CORONARY SPASM.

Sphygmomanometer   The apparatus used with a stethoscope to measure blood pressure.

Static exercise   Contrasted to aerobic, cardiovascular or
C.V. or DYNAMIC EXERCISE, static exercise is sporadic, like
lifting weights or chopping wood, and does not sustain
a heart rate at a higher level for a beneficial length of
time.

Statins   A group of drugs that, taken orally, lowers levels
of CHOLESTEROL and TRIGLYCERIDES in the blood, sometimes very dramatically. The most commonly used ones
are: LOVASTATIN, sold under the brand name MEVACOR
(Merck); PRAVASTATIN, brand name PRAVACHOL (Bristol-
Myers Squibb); SIMVASTATIN, sold as ZOCOR (Merck); and
FLUVASTATIN, sold as LESCOL (Sandoz). They are more
technically HMG-COA REDUCTASE INHIBITORS and block

an enzyme essential to the body's manufacture of CHOLESTEROL.

Stenosis The narrowing of a blood vessel or valve caused by disease or blockage.

Stent A structure or mechanism placed inside a collapsed blood vessel to support it from within, specifically after a failed ANGIOPLASTY; a stainless-steel coil is currently in occasional use.

Sternotomy, median The surgical approach to the heart from the front, through the breastbone.

Sternum The breastbone.

Stress A strain or tension put on the body or mind by physical or emotional demands or chemical agents; a very real, but unquantifiable, risk factor in heart disease.

Stress test See EXERCISE EKG.

Subclavian vein The continuation of the axillary vein that runs from the outer border of the first rib to the inner end of the clavicle or collarbone.

Swan-Ganz catheter A device used to record and monitor temperature and pressure in the pulmonary artery.

Systole The part of the heart's normal cycle when the ventricles contract, creating systolic pressure.

Tachycardia An abnormally fast heartbeat.

Teboroxime A radioactive tracer used similarly to SESTAMIBI or THALLIUM in STRESS TESTS.

Thallium stress test An EXERCISE EKG to which is added an intravenous injection of a solution containing a radioactive isotope of the element thallium. A scanning X-ray camera then reveals the areas of the heart with inadequate blood and oxygen supply, since they will absorb less thallium than the better supplied areas.

Thoracic artery See INTERNAL THORACIC ARTERY.

Thrombosis   The formation of a blood clot or THROMBUS within a blood vessel or the heart itself.

Thromboxane   A substance produced in the body that damages arterial wall; its production is suppressed by OMEGA-3 FATTY ACIDS.

Thrombus   A blood clot.

TOMHS   Treatment Of Mild Hypertension Study, a study that tracked 902 people with mild hypertension (DIASTOLIC pressure between 90 and 99) over five years and demonstrated that any of five standard blood pressure–lowering drugs was effective and beneficial and that taking such medication reduced the risk of stroke or heart attack by 32 percent.

Trans fatty acids   See ACIDS, TRANS FATTY.

Trans-myocardial revascularization   An experimental method of providing a new blood supply *within* the heart by piercing the heart itself with large numbers of laser beam pulses, creating many tiny interior channels where blood can circulate. The entrance and exit holes made by the beams are sufficiently small as to be self-closing and the blood supply is from the heart itself.

Tricuspid valve   In the heart, the VALVE between the right ATRIUM and right VENTRICLE.

Triglycerides   Molecules formed of three fatty acid molecules combined with glycerol; they are formed from the products of digestion and are the form in which fat is stored in the body.

Ultrasound   See ECHOCARDIOGRAM.

Valve   In the heart, a two-lobed (bicuspid) or three-lobed (tricuspid) structure between one compartment or vessel and another and through which blood is able to flow in only one direction.

Vascular disease   Any disease of the blood vessels, particularly CORONARY HEART or ARTERY DISEASE.

Vasodilator   A drug used to increase the interior diameter of a blood vessel.

Veins   Vessels through which deoxygenated blood passes from the body back to the heart and lungs.

Vena(e) cava(e)   The two large veins through which deoxygenated blood passes from the body into the right ATRIUM of the heart; the *inferior* vena cava conveys blood from the body below the diaphragm, and the *superior* vena cava conveys blood from the upper body.

Ventricle   One of the two lower chambers in the heart whose function is to pump blood. The *right* ventricle receives deoxygenated blood from the sequence body—VENAE CAVAE, right ATRIUM—and pumps it through the pulmonary artery into the lungs; the *left* ventricle receives oxygenated blood from the sequence lungs—pulmonary vein, left atrium—and pumps it through the AORTA back to the body.

Ventricular fibrillation   See FIBRILLATION.

Venule   A minute blood vessel that draws blood from capillaries and joins with others to form a VEIN.

Vessel   The collective term for both veins and arteries, the tubes that bear blood to and from the heart.

VLDL   Very Low Density Lipoprotein, the protein used by the liver to manufacture LDL, or low density lipoprotein, and the transporter of TRIGLYCERIDES.

Zocor   The brand name of SIMVASTATIN; see STATINS.

Suggested Reading

As you might imagine, the literature devoted to coronary artery disease is vast indeed, most of it highly technical. Of the comparatively few books written for the layman, most were written by surgeons or cardiologists with the help of professional writers, and these books seem to me to be like advice about pregnancy from male physicians. In any event, here are a few specific recommendations: Dr. Legato's book for women is *the* book for this specific audience; Dr. Phibbs's book is excellent for general information about the heart and many of its ailments; Green, Singh, and Sosa is the great technical work and will tell you all there is to know about the surgical techniques; and Dean Ornish's book is must reading for anyone at risk for heart disease.

Arthur Fisher, *The Healthy Heart.* Alexandria, Va: Time-Life Books, 1981.

George E. Green, M.D., Ram N. Singh, M.D., and J. A. Sosa, M.D., *Surgical Revascularization of the Heart: The Internal Thoracic Arteries.* New York and Tokyo: Igaku-Shoin Medical Publishers, 1991.

Jonathan L. Halperin, M.D., and Richard Levine, *Bypass.* Tucson, Ariz.: The Body Press, 1987.

Harvard Health Letter. Cambridge, Mass.: Harvard University. Published monthly.

Harvard Heart Letter. Cambridge, Mass.: Harvard University. Published monthly.

Steve G. Hubbard, M.D., and Gary Ferguson, *Recovering from Coronary Bypass Surgery.* New York: HarperPaperbacks, 1992.

Learning to Live With Angina. Boston, Mass.: Medicine in the Public Interest, 1981.

Learning to Live With Coronary Artery Disease. Boston, Mass.: Medicine in the Public Interest, 1993.

Marianne J. Legato, M.D., and Carol Colman, *The Female Heart.* New York: Simon and Schuster, 1991.

Mayo Clinic Heart Book, Michael D. McGoon. New York: William Morrow, 1993.

Dean Ornish, M.D., *Dr. Dean Ornish's Program for Reversing Heart Disease.* New York: Random House, 1990.

Brendan Phibbs, M.D., *The Human Heart.* New York: New American Library, 1982.

The Surgeon General's Report on Nutrition and Health. Rocklin, Calif.: Prima Publishing and Communications, 1988.

Yale University School of Medicine Heart Book. Barry L. Zaret, M.D., Marvin Moser, M.D., and Lawrence S. Cohen, M.D. New York: Hearst Books, 1992.

There are many, many cookbooks for heart-healthy diets and it is difficult to choose among them. A particularly good one, though, is:

Gail L. Becker, *Heart Smart.* New York: Pocket Books, 1987.

Index